"*Super Natural Home* seeks out the silent violence—i.e., toxins—in and around the place where you spend most of your time, awake and asleep. . . It's required for anyone with a home and a healthy desire to

—RALPH NADER, LAWYER AND

"Making simple changes can often have a profoun family's health but also on the planet. Beth Gree creating a practical resource that will let you kno. .... these changes are and how to easily implement them."

—JOSEPH MERCOLA, DO, FOUNDER OF MERCOLA.COM

"In a world where we are overexposed to thousands of dangerous toxic chemicals, education is the key. *Super Natural Home* provides vital information for anyone interested in reducing their chemical exposure."

—DAN JACOBSON, LEGISLATIVE DIRECTOR,
ENVIRONMENT CALIFORNIA

"*Super Natural Home* offers important information on how to stay healthy along with practical, easy tips that are backed by scientific research. Every household should have this book on hand."

—MARCI SHIMOFF, NEW YORK TIMES BEST-SELLING AUTHOR,
HAPPY FOR NO REASON AND CHICKEN SOUP FOR THE
WOMAN'S SOUL

"Beth Greer is a knowledgeable expert, and every reader will benefit from the insightful instructions and questions she offers that empower us to change the way we live for ourselves and future generations."

—LYNNE TWIST, PRESIDENT, SOUL OF MONEY INSTITUTE, AND
CO-FOUNDER, THE PACHAMAMA ALLIANCE

"I love this book! It gives a unique blend of the author's personal experience as well as cutting-edge research to enlighten us on how our environment impacts our health. I highly recommend it."

—CATHERINE OXENBERG, AWARD-WINNING
ACTRESS AND MOTHER OF FIVE

"Beth Greer is a correspondent on the front lines who leaves no stone unturned in her search for emerging news of crucial and timely relevance to wellness in today's changing environment. I am eternally grateful to her as a resource for my family, my patients, and the entire globe. Thank you, Super Natural Mom!"

—MICHELLE VENEZIANO, DO, FAMILY PRACTICE PHYSICIAN,
MILL VALLEY, CALIFORNIA

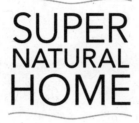

SUPER
NATURAL
HOME

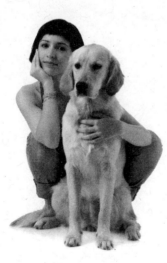

SUPER
NATURAL
HOME

Improve Your Health, Home, and Planet— One Room at a Time

BETH GREER
Super Natural Mom™

RODALE

Rodale books may be purchased for business or promotional use or for special sales. For information, please write to:
Special Markets Department, Rodale Inc., 733 Third Avenue, New York, NY 10017
Printed in the United States of America
Rodale Inc. makes every effort to use acid-free ♾, recycled paper ♻.

Book design by Christina Gaugler

Library of Congress Cataloging-in-Publication Data

Greer, Beth.
    Super natural home : improve your health, home, and planet one room at a time / Beth Greer, Super Natural Mom.
        p.   cm.
    Includes index.
    ISBN-13: 978–1–60529–981–5 paperback
    ISBN-10: 1–60529–981–2 paperback
    1. Holistic medicine.   2. Alternative lifestyles.   I. Title.
R733.G735   2009
615.9'02—dc22   2008054574

Distributed to the trade by Macmillan

2   4   6   8   10   9   7   5   3   1   paperback

We inspire and enable people to improve their lives and the world around them
For more of our products visit **rodalestore.com** or call 800-848-4735

For my Grandma Bertha

CONTENTS

Section I: What Goes *in* You: How to Eliminate Exposure to Toxic Chemicals in Your Food and Drinking Water

Section II: What Goes *on* You: How to Choose Safe Cosmetics and Body Care Products

Section III: What *Surrounds* You: How to Minimize Indoor Air Pollution in Your Home Environment

Section IV: Supporting Information

FOREWORD

WAY BACK IN 2004, I had this very simple idea for a book that I took to my publisher. I said green living can also be gorgeous living. It doesn't have to mean sacrificing style or convenience or having a wonderful life. It's taking natural living—beyond straw bale houses and Birkenstock-lined hallways—up a notch. It's *super* natural living! Unfortunately, this fantastic, futuristic, this-is-how-we're-all-going-to-live idea was met with stares and finally a blunt question: Did I want to write a book about the supernatural life of wizardry, ghosts, and goblins? So, I moved on and never wrote that book.

Flash forward several years, and it doesn't take much to realize that green living is on everyone's mind today. You turn on the TV to watch green renovation makeover shows, or flip through a special "green" issue of a popular magazine or even watch *An Inconvenient Truth*. Stroll through popular stores like Lowe's and JCPenney (where I am their Green Living Partner) and you'll find myriad eco-friendly products at everyday low prices. With this flood of green, some might think going eco-friendly is trendy! It's hip! It's cool! And I say I hope it's anything but that.

The word "trendy" scares me because to me it means something that's very en vogue one moment and totally out the next (read: Ugg boots). What I do think is happening is a cultural shift, a seismic move in the way we live and think about everyday living. And I can pinpoint the actual moment our country shifted from naysayer to treehugger: when gas prices hit the roof. When people realized their wasteful habits affected their wallets, everything changed. Hybrids went from concept car to hottest ride. And pretty soon, we started to re-evaluate everything else in our lives to conserve resources and save money, too.

Now with the publication of Beth Greer's fantastic book *Super Natural Home*, not only am I excited for this fabulous guide to living a healthy and green life, but I feel redeemed. I had a hunch several years ago that there were many people—like myself and Beth—who felt the world of natural living needed a facelift. This book is what I consider a refresher of what we know and where we need to go to live a greener and healthier life. Sure, we all know that compact fluorescent light bulbs are good for the planet since they're energy efficient and last up to eight times longer than antiquated incandescent bulbs. But what else should we be doing in our homes that we're neglecting or just haven't thought about changing? In *Super Natural Home*, Beth takes you step by step, room by room to make it easy and almost delightful to do.

I get thousands of questions from people who say they feel overwhelmed by the process of going green. So, I always say to start with Just One Thing. Do just one thing each day and over time your actions accumulatively build up to something great and truly impactful. By picking up Beth's new book, you're one step closer to doing just one great thing for your home.

–Danny Seo
Environmental lifestyle expert and Living Green
editor for *Better Homes and Gardens*

ACKNOWLEDGMENTS

THIS BOOK IS A WORK OF SYNTHESIS, based on the research and insights of many in the fields of food, environmental toxins, and health. In educating myself on these issues, I've been inspired and enlightened by people like Deepak Chopra, who taught me that the body is a self-healing organism; Michael Pollan, for opening my eyes to how our food is produced, in his 2002 *New York Times Magazine* article "Power Steer," and his subsequent books and articles, which changed the way I eat; Dr. Devra Davis, for her groundbreaking research on cancer and environmental toxins; Eric Schlosser, for the insights I gained from reading his book *Fast Food Nation*; Dr. Joseph Mercola, for his wealth of knowledge on food and nutrition; Lynne Twist, for her passion for the planet and for sharing her thoughts about shopping with consciousness; Debra Lynn Dadd, consumer advocate, for her pioneering work in the field of nontoxic and natural products; as well as the amazing daily newsfeeds from naturalnews.com and the nonprofit organization Environmental Health Sciences.

A deep debt of gratitude goes to the following people as well:

Jody Weiss, for being my best cheerleader and dear friend, who encouraged me to write my very first newspaper column. Her loving nature, fierce passion for what she does, and intense good will are an inspiration to me and to women everywhere.

Brenda Wade, Heidi Wise, and Karen Leland, for their benevolently beautiful advice and guidance.

Alex Mandossian, marketing guru, for his generous and brilliant coaching.

Eric Harr, humanitarian and professional athlete, for his guidance and amazing contribution.

Bill Zanker, founder of the Learning Annex, for his coaching, encouragement, incredible energy, and enthusiastic support.

Carol Goodman, for her gracious guidance, sensible advice, and generous counsel.

Lynette Evans, editor of the Home Section of the *San Francisco Chronicle*, who hired me to write columns that sparked the idea for this book.

Jennifer Jerde, who was extremely generous with design advice, and her staff, and for introducing me to Aaron Cruse, who designed my unique and beautiful logo. .

Carolyn and Allan Nation, for introducing me to Michael Pollan and for being so supportive of my work.

Warren Farrell, for encouraging me to attend the Book Expo America event, where I connected with Susan Berg at Rodale.

Jayme Canton, Paul Gilbert, and Jennifer Machiorlatti, for their help in formulating my ideas for the book at its inception.

Randy Martin, my biggest fan, who cheered me on, every step of the way, as well as my other phenomenal friends who have given me love, encouragement, guidance, and support: Brenda Wade and Gerald Harris, Shelly and Morty Lefkoe, Janet Atwood, Marci Shimoff, Beth DeWoody, Jain Wager and my Bolinas Tribe, Michael Lutin, Lily Kanter, Deborah Luster, Tom Koenig, Maryanne Comaroto, Joanne Zippel, Joyce Shank, Marcia Wieder, Adi Gorel, Barry and Marti Fischer, Diane Valentine, Sandi Padnos, Flora Bernard, Andy Rostolder, Bunny Sandrock, Dianne Morrison, Beverly Parenti, Howard Nemerov, Roy Forest, Ariel Jordan, Malcolm MacDonald, Susanne Paynovich, Caral Newman, Marianne Stefancic, Raz and Liza Ingrasci, Anat Baniel, Betsy Rosenberg, Meg Jordan, and Dick Bolles.

I would also like to thank my influential journalism teachers at New York University, Graduate School of Arts and Sciences—Helen Epstein, Teri Schultz, Mitchell Stephens, and Jesse Kornbluth, who helped me hone my writing skills as well as encourage me to look at the world with a distinctive point of view.

Richard Unger, for helping me clarify my life's purpose as a writer, and Dr. Heidi Dulay, for giving me the opportunity to teach what I know.

Kathi Altman, for giving me a structure to tap into my own rhythm, and express myself with authenticity; Marilyn Graman and Maureen Walsh, for teaching me how to build a nurturing relationship with my inner self; and Alon MacCarthy, for being my spiritual mentor and cheerleader.

Marc Weill, for helping me rid my body of my tumor and educating me about the importance of detoxifying from the chemicals in our bodies; and Dr. Ellen Cutler, for keeping me radiantly healthy.

I offer deep thanks to Bonnie Solow, my literary agent and dear friend, who offered invaluable strategic guidance and support. Susan Berg, my editor at Rodale, for bringing her years of experience to each page and making this book a reality. Kristin Loberg, who helped me throughout the entire writing process with encouragement and great editorial skill, as well as a delightful, easy working style; and Steven Weinberg, for his impeccable legal counsel and great sense of humor.

Special thanks to Jake, my poodle buddy, who made sure I took him for walks in nature where I could clear my head and listen to my inner guidance.

To Esther, Bertha's daughter and my Mom, for her unconditional love, for always believing in me, and for being the role model of health and fitness in her nineties.

To Casey, my daughter, who amazes me daily with her creativity, energy, and wisdom, and for teaching me how to be more playful.

And finally, Stephen Seligman, my superhero, husband, anchor, and favorite person of all time, for his continuous support, humor, guidance, and cut-to-the-chase advice. His flexibility in accommodating my writing schedule and for making sure our kitchen was always well stocked with organic produce were invaluable to me. Almost 20 years of living together, working together, and growing together; this book wouldn't exist without his presence in my life.

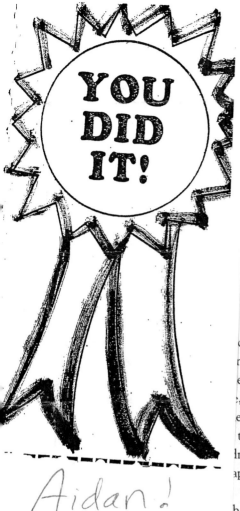

UCTION

Your Home
in a Toxic World

e first step."

— CHINESE PROVERB

der, was my inspiration for becoming a
nnenbaum, she grew up in Austria, and in
erica via Ellis Island. She was generous,
, and robustly healthy, and she created a
er 94 years on this planet. Grandma never
to the market several times a week. Like
In't waste money. Instead, she reused "tin"
aper, and reminded me to "close the lights"

he lived simply and made do with very lit-
outside to dry in the sunlight and cleaned
the floors and windows ly furnished Brooklyn apartment with vinegar and water. She "washed" her teeth with a natural tooth powder, and made
her own clothes using a black Singer sewing machine powered by a simple foot
pedal instead of electricity.

My grandmother—who had beautiful skin and clear gray-green eyes—
wore no make-up. And she never used canned food; "always fresh" was her
motto. She'd shop at the local butcher or fish market and pick out fresh chicken
or fish for dinner. She cooked three meals a day from scratch, always with fresh
fruit and vegetables, and more often than not homemade bread.

How times have changed! Today most of us eat meals that come from a

Aidan !

package, can, or box. We use makeup, body care, and cleaning products that contain complex chemical compounds we can hardly pronounce, let alone understand. We live in a world more complicated, polluted, and risky to our environment and personal health than my grandmother could have ever imagined. Hundreds of chemicals in our food, cosmetics, cookware, and furniture have been banned in countries around the world but are available here in the United States without warning labels. Without regulation by our government, it falls on us as consumers to watch out for ourselves and our families.

If you're like most people, a little voice inside your head has probably been telling you for a while that it's time to get back to a more natural way of living and take a more serious look at the toxins in your everyday life. Even so, you may feel confused about the simple, practical things you can do to minimize your exposure and maximize not only your health but also your contribution to a cleaner planet. You might feel bombarded by conflicting information and not have a clear understanding of what's harmful and what's not. For example: Do all nonstick pans emit harmful chemicals? Do artificial sweeteners cause cancer?

Before we get to those answers, I want to first congratulate you for picking up this book. The material in it has the potential to alter your life forever. After reading *Super Natural Home* you will know how to transform your house into a safe haven from the chemicals you're exposed to daily. This book will dispel commonly held myths; offer insights into what makes certain foods, body care products, household cleaners, cookware, and furniture toxic; and paint a truthful, albeit alarming, picture of our daily world. This picture is meant not to frighten you but instead to arm you with a newfound awareness that will bring you peace of mind, along with the knowledge you need to feel safe. For every worrisome statistic or fact that you learn, you'll find at least one antidote or easy idea to lessen its impact in your life.

I commend you for the action you're taking just by reading these pages, which I hope will motivate and inspire you to make small shifts in what you've already been doing. The tips and strategies I share here are doable, economical, and life changing. Make a promise to yourself to read this book all the way through. My promise back to you is that you will feel empowered instead of frightened and that you will have a healthier, more vibrant tomorrow. We all have the opportunity to access both the old world tradition of my grandmother's time and the new-world conveniences of modern life. We have more choices than my grandmother did for living healthy—we simply have to *choose* the best of both worlds.

INTRODUCTION

Transform Your Home
into a Safe Haven in a Toxic World

"A long journey begins with the first step."

— CHINESE PROVERB

MY GRANDMA, Bertha Rostolder, was my inspiration for becoming a Super Natural Mom. Born Bluma Tannenbaum, she grew up in Austria, and in 1905, at age 16, immigrated to America via Ellis Island. She was generous, kind, smart, hard-working, intuitive, and robustly healthy, and she created a very small carbon footprint during her 94 years on this planet. Grandma never learned to drive and so she walked to the market several times a week. Like many immigrants of her era, she didn't waste money. Instead, she reused "tin" foil, used cloth napkins instead of paper, and reminded me to "close the lights" when leaving a room.

During the Great Depression she lived simply and made do with very little. She hung her laundry on a line outside to dry in the sunlight and cleaned the floors and windows of her simply furnished Brooklyn apartment with vinegar and water. She "washed" her teeth with a natural tooth powder, and made her own clothes using a black Singer sewing machine powered by a simple foot pedal instead of electricity.

My grandmother—who had beautiful skin and clear gray-green eyes—wore no make-up. And she never used canned food; "always fresh" was her motto. She'd shop at the local butcher or fish market and pick out fresh chicken or fish for dinner. She cooked three meals a day from scratch, always with fresh fruit and vegetables, and more often than not homemade bread.

How times have changed! Today most of us eat meals that come from a package, can, or box. We use makeup, body care, and cleaning products that contain complex chemical compounds we can hardly pronounce, let alone understand. We live in a world more complicated, polluted, and risky to our environment and personal health than my grandmother could have ever imagined. Hundreds of chemicals in our food, cosmetics, cookware, and furniture have been banned in countries around the world but are available here in the United States without warning labels. Without regulation by our government, it falls on us as consumers to watch out for ourselves and our families.

If you're like most people, a little voice inside your head has probably been telling you for a while that it's time to get back to a more natural way of living and take a more serious look at the toxins in your everyday life. Even so, you may feel confused about the simple, practical things you can do to minimize your exposure and maximize not only your health but also your contribution to a cleaner planet. You might feel bombarded by conflicting information and not have a clear understanding of what's harmful and what's not. For example: Do all nonstick pans emit harmful chemicals? Do artificial sweeteners cause cancer?

Before we get to those answers, I want to first congratulate you for picking up this book. The material in it has the potential to alter your life forever. After reading *Super Natural Home* you will know how to transform your house into a safe haven from the chemicals you're exposed to daily. This book will dispel commonly held myths; offer insights into what makes certain foods, body care products, household cleaners, cookware, and furniture toxic; and paint a truthful, albeit alarming, picture of our daily world. This picture is meant not to frighten you but instead to arm you with a newfound awareness that will bring you peace of mind, along with the knowledge you need to feel safe. For every worrisome statistic or fact that you learn, you'll find at least one antidote or easy idea to lessen its impact in your life.

I commend you for the action you're taking just by reading these pages, which I hope will motivate and inspire you to make small shifts in what you've already been doing. The tips and strategies I share here are doable, economical, and life changing. Make a promise to yourself to read this book all the way through. My promise back to you is that you will feel empowered instead of frightened and that you will have a healthier, more vibrant tomorrow. We all have the opportunity to access both the old world tradition of my grandmother's time and the new-world conveniences of modern life. We have more choices than my grandmother did for living healthy—we simply have to *choose* the best of both worlds.

A SNAPSHOT OF STATISTICS

On an average day you're exposed to hundreds, maybe thousands of chemicals . . . from the additives in your food and personal care products to things you come in contact with, such as your mattress or couch or even the paint on your walls. Green groups and scientists are releasing frightening studies about discovering chemical toxins in powdered milk, plastic toys, carpeting, and lipstick. You hear reports almost daily with gloomy statistics like these:

- According to a 2007 front-page story in the *Los Angeles Times*, an article in the journal *Cancer* concluded that more than 200 chemicals—many found in everyday consumer products—cause breast cancer in animals. (Researchers concur that reducing exposure to these compounds could prevent the disease in humans.)

- The Environmental Protection Agency reports that the average US home produces twice as many greenhouse emissions as a single car, and the air inside our homes can be five to 100 times more polluted than the air outside because of the toxic fumes emanating from our household cleaners, carpeting, and wallpaper.

- The cosmetics industry is unregulated by the government, which means that manufacturers of makeup, lotions, deodorants, and mouthwashes can put almost anything they want into their products—without necessarily telling you everything on the label.

- According to the World Health Organization, every day, nine of 10 American children between ages 6 months and 5 years are exposed to combinations of 13 different organophosphate insecticides in the foods they eat.

Learning about the links between the environment and our health can feel confusing and scary. You care, but you might think, "I can't do anything about the chemicals in our environment," or "I really don't see how I can make a difference."

Well, what if I told you that making small, simple changes in your everyday routine could have a huge impact on your health and well-being, and even the health of our planet? I will share with you what motivated me to start making changes in my life.

CLEANING UP MY ACT

I discovered I had a tumor in my chest. Until then, I thought I was leading a "healthy" life. I wasn't overweight, I exercised a few times a week, and I meditated. I didn't smoke, rarely drank, and ate food that I considered to be nourishing. I was, however, very stressed.

For the previous 10 years, I had been running a business with my husband. The business was The Learning Annex, an adult education school that we expanded from one location to six cities across the United States and Canada. I felt like an acrobat spinning plates on long sticks, running back and forth, constantly monitoring each plate to ensure it was spinning at a good rate. Once a plate would wobble, it would surely fall and break. My schools were like the plates, and I made sure that each school was as wobble-free as possible.

Because of my hectic schedule, I ate out regularly and often had energy bars for breakfast or lunch. Sound familiar? I think everyone operates in this high-wire mode more than once in a while.

We had adopted a baby 4 years earlier, and I was doing my best to manage as a working mom and maintain a happy marriage. Imagine spending the whole day—all week long—running a business with your spouse and then trying to feel sexy toward one another at night. It was nearly impossible! We sought couples counseling and devised strategies to assist us with the stress. One was not to talk business after 10:30 at night unless we both agreed on it. Well, that didn't really work. Invariably one of us would suddenly blurt something out just as we were falling asleep. That was me in 2001. I was 49 years old, working nonstop, then taking 2 weeks off for a vacation—during which I obsessed about my business the whole time. I was orchestrating events with thousands of people in attendance who came to see the spiritual and business gurus of our time, as well as the motivational experts who spoke about balance—something I was lacking. I was overseeing a staff, and writing copy or editing someone else's for the catalogs we printed each month. I was constantly coming up with new course ideas because if the classes weren't fresh, then people, I believed, wouldn't sign up and our business would fail.

It's no wonder my shoulder started to hurt! I went to a chiropractor, who suggested I get an MRI because his treatments weren't helping my pain, which was now traveling down my arm into my hand. The MRI showed a large mass (5 cm) in my chest. What? Me? This can't be happening to me! I ate fruits and vegetables and felt fine! The radiologist wrote on the report that it was possibly breast cancer. That's when the pain suddenly intensified.

After a mammogram ruled out breast cancer (whew!), I had a CT scan and biopsy of the mass that was in my chest cavity. Thank goodness it was benign, with no trace of cancer cells. I saw three different thoracic surgeons at three different San Francisco hospitals, each with a different idea about how to remove the tumor. One told me he would make an incision under my collar bone, the next wanted to go in from my armpit, and the third wanted to cut me on my back and remove one of my ribs in order to reach the tumor. I then sought the advice of a neurosurgeon, who told me to put off having surgery as long as I could bear the pain; there were so many nerves in that area of the body that a surgical procedure would put me at "high risk" for losing feeling in my fingers permanently.

My head was spinning and the pain was worsening. The mass was pressing on the brachial plexus, a bundle of nerves that runs down the arm. By chance, I had made arrangements months earlier to fly down to San Diego and spend a week with a friend of mine at the Optimum Health Institute (OHI). Our plan was to get away and chill out at what I thought was a retreat center. I was unaware that OHI was actually a place to detoxify the body with diet, fasting, cleansing, and exercise; to quiet the mind with journaling and meditation; and to strengthen the spirit with study, prayer, and celebration. It turned out to be the perfect place for me to start my healing journey.

After the fourth day of juice fasting and learning destressing techniques in the OHI program, I noticed that I no longer needed a pill to help me to sleep at night because the pain was diminishing. I discovered that the body is a self-healing organism if we just get out of its way and don't gunk it up with bad food and stress. When I arrived home a week later, I decided to continue to eat a raw-food diet, which consisted of fruits, vegetables, and nuts, until my pain was completely gone. In addition, I sought the help of a naturopath in San Francisco named Marc Weill. He told me that he believed my lymph nodes had gotten clogged and had formed a mass because of toxins in my bloodstream. He helped me to continue to detoxify my body by using special supplements and drinking raw vegetable juices as well as other techniques to get the lymph moving.

During this period, I decided to expand my cleanse from the inside out. I became conscious not only of what I was eating and drinking but also of what I was putting on my skin and what was surrounding me. I bought nontoxic household cleaners; I found new natural makeup; I replaced my old mattress with a new one that contained no flame retardants or polyester, which are known carcinogens. Six months after my initial diagnosis, in May 2002, on my

50th birthday, the pain was so slight that I started to introduce cooked food again. By the end of the month the pain was completely gone. I had another CT scan and the mass had disappeared!

Within 2 months of that scan, my husband and I decided to sell our business. And then I started to write—first about other people who have healed themselves using alternative means, and then about how each of us has the ability to heal. And now I'm writing to let you know how to protect yourself. Don't wait until you get sick! Fix things now in your immediate environment and prevent a potential health crisis from occurring.

FROM OVERWHELMED TO AWARENESS AND ACTION!

This book, if you follow my suggestions, will arm you with empowering and accurate information so you can start to make wise lifestyle choices from the inside out. I'm not a doctor, nutritionist, or scientist, and this book is not intended as a cure for illness. Rather, I'm a journalist and holistic health advocate who has done extensive research on the subject and whose sizable tumor was eliminated without drugs or surgery. My goal is to guide you by introducing you to information and providing you with practical suggestions and manageable solutions that are easy and inexpensive and that have the most impact on creating a green, toxin-free life. I will also offer scientific research to validate what I present in this book.

To begin, I've put together a 20-question quiz (I call it the Super Natural Home Quiz) that will help you assess where, when, and how often you may be exposed to toxins in your daily routine. It's important to scrutinize what you're currently burdened with over the course of the day.

I want you to get curious about what's in your food (even where it's grown); what's in your makeup, deodorant, soap, and shampoo, and who's regulating the safety of these products; and how the cookware, fabrics, and furniture you come in contact with can also affect your health. You will gain insight into the choices you've already made, and from there you can begin the process of making new choices. This quiz will jumpstart your awareness and essentially prime you for the journey you will take with me.

The book is then broken down into four parts. In Section I, What Goes in You: How to Eliminate Exposure to Toxic Chemicals in Your Food and Drinking Water, you'll learn about the Fearsome 5 Things to Avoid. These are things you swallow that can zap your energy and make you sick. I'll teach you how to read labels, what questions to ask yourself when shopping, what you should know about plastic drinking bottles, and which toxic chemicals to avoid. You'll learn why it's important to eliminate pesticides, food additives such as MSG, trans fats and artificial sweeteners, factory-farmed and genetically modified foods, and unfiltered tap water from your diet.

In Section II, What Goes *on* You: How to Choose Safe Cosmetics and Body Care Products, you'll learn what to look for in safe products, how to do research on your own, and how to find the best substitutes for what you're using now. In Section III, What *Surrounds* You: How to Minimize Indoor Air Pollution in Your Home Environment, you will start taking control of the everyday things you come in contact with in your environment. You'll discover the best cleaning products; the safest cookware; and how to choose furnishings, paint, and flooring for every room in your home. You can then begin to make changes as your budget allows. And, speaking of budgets, you'll be surprised to discover that in many instances nontoxic products won't cost you more than what you're already using.

As a bonus, you will learn how to take Super Natural Home consciousness on the road when you eat at restaurants, stay in hotels, go on vacation, or send your kids to school or summer camp, as well as additional strategies to optimize your health and well-being.

Finally, Section IV, Supporting Information: Recommended Resources, will help provide you with highly informative books, Web sites, and blogs, and will help you find the best green, sustainable, nontoxic products as well as holistic practitioners who can help you remove toxins that have accumulated in your body. (Please note that the product suggestions in this book are meant to be examples of what is available and not a complete listing.)

By easily upgrading and eliminating toxins in each room of your house, you can experience the pleasure of helping reduce your footprint on the planet as well as enhancing your health and well-being. You'll find that the slight

"We know humans are exposed to mixtures [of chemicals], and studying mixtures is very difficult. We will never have the whole picture, and it will take many, many years to collect epidemiological evidence, so we should take some preventive measures now."

—ANA SOTO, MD, a professor of cell biology at Tufts University who specializes in the cellular origins of cancer and the effects of hormone-disrupting contaminants lifestyle shifts you make are rewarding not only to your home but to your body and spirit as well. In my experience, as I became aware of and eliminated the "bad" stuff in my foods and personal care products, my stamina and energy improved dramatically.

Vitality is within each of us. To connect with it, we first must understand that it is suppressed when our bodies are fighting off toxins. Chemicals are invisible (you can't see them on a piece of fruit or in carpet, nail polish, or soap), but they can wreak havoc on our immune systems.

Studies are coming out frequently about how everyday chemicals in our bodies are resulting in health problems such as learning disabilities, autism, cancer, and infertility. Often, the impact of chemicals doesn't show up for decades—as with tobacco, for example. What remains unclear is what happens inside our bodies when we come into contact with different chemicals from lots of different sources. No one has done research on the different types of interactions that can occur when chemicals combine. What are the risks for us and our children?

Don't wait to find out! You can do something right now, right in your own home. I guarantee that if you follow the advice in the following pages, you will be surprised at how easy some of the adjustments are to make and how quickly their benefits can be felt. We all deserve to feel and be as healthy and vital as possible. The choice is yours.

Now, let's take the Super Natural Home Quiz!

SUPER NATURAL HOME QUIZ

Take an Inventory of Your Daily Exposure to Dangerous Chemicals

"You've got bad eating habits if you use a grocery cart in 7-Eleven."

— DENNIS MILLER

WHETHER WE LIVE in an old or a new home or apartment, it can be shocking to realize how we expose ourselves to toxic chemicals on a daily basis. Sometimes we take clean to an extreme and unwittingly buy disinfectants and cleansers that can compromise our health and well-being. Or we're not aware of the hidden additives in our food, or the effects of the invisible gasses that are released from plastics or flame retardants in our furniture.

In this quiz we're going to take a look at every room in your home, from the foods (and containers) inside your fridge and pantry, to the bottles lining your sinks and shower stalls, to the furniture and accessories with which you come into daily contact. As you move from room to room, let your eyes, your nose, and even your intuition be your guide.

START THE QUIZ

Grab a pen or pencil and a notebook. Ask your children and spouse to join you. It can be fun and educational for them as well. I promise this will be worth your time. Start by writing down the date you take this quiz. The results will help you identify and focus on areas needing improvement. You can take the quiz again in 6 months, after you've made positive changes, to see how well you're doing.

I'm going to ask you to take a close look at what you're buying and why. This is an exercise that will provide insight into your choices so you can get a sense of just how often you are exposed to chemicals in your home. Don't worry! Once you see the choices you've made, you can start making new choices that will enhance your well-being, keep you and your family healthy, and even improve the health of the planet. And I'm going to show you how to do just that step by step. It's easier than you think, and the rewards are infinite. Let's get started.

The Kitchen, Pantry, and Refrigerator:

1. **Does the food you eat contain pesticides?**

    ☐ Yes   ☐ No   ☐ Don't know

    Hint: If the food in question is not labeled organic or not grown on a local farm, it almost certainly will contain pesticides.

    Problem: Pesticides are designed to kill, and are toxic to us and the environment. They are known to harm the human neurologic system and to deplete the Earth's protective ozone layer, leading to more skin cancer.

    Solution: See Chapter 1

2. **Does the food you eat contain growth hormones?**

    ☐ Yes   ☐ No   ☐ Don't know

    Hint: If the meat or poultry isn't organic or "grass-fed" (raised on pasture), or your milk pro ducts aren't labeled organic, they probably contain growth hormones. (Later on, I'll share what this could mean from a biological standpoint.)

    Problem: As many as two-thirds of cattle raised in the United States are injected with rBGH (recombinant bovine growth hormone) to make them produce more milk. The milk is shipped throughout the country, added to products such as cream, cheese, yogurt, and baked goods, but never labeled as such.

    Solution: See Chapter 3

3. **Do your beverages contain artificial sweeteners?**

☐ Yes ☐ No ☐ Don't know

Hint: All "diet" soda contains artificial sweeteners. The same goes for foods and other beverages labeled with the words "diet, "lite," "sugarless," or "no sugar." Lots of low-calorie snacks are marketed as such because they swap out the real thing for artificial sugars. Look for names such as NutraSweet, Sweet'n Low, Equal, sucralose, and aspartame.

Problem: Artificial sweeteners are known hazards. Aspartame, considered a ticking time bomb by scientists, may actually stimulate appetite and bring on a craving for carbohydrates. In addition, aspartame contains methanol, which the body breaks down into formaldehyde. (Formaldehyde is one of the main substances pumped into a dead body during the embalming process!)

Solution: See Chapter 2

4. **Does your food or beverages contain high-fructose corn syrup?**

☐ Yes ☐ No ☐ Don't know

Hint: Most brands of soda, even natural ones, are sweetened mainly with high-fructose corn syrup (HFCS), the product of a complex industrial process in which starch is extracted from corn and converted into glucose and fructose. HFCS is also ubiquitous in condiments, snacks, and "sugary" beverages, even if those drinks are not classified as "soda." You'll find it listed under ingredients.

Problem: Researchers agree that HFCS is a major contributor to Americans' calorie intake and a significant cause of overweight and obesity—a prime risk factor for type 2 diabetes, which is on the rise.

Solution: See Chapter 2

5. **Do you use Teflon-coated or other nonstick cookware?**

☐ Yes ☐ No ☐ Don't know

Hint: Almost all brands of nonstick cookware have a toxic coating.

Problem: Most nonstick cookware gives off odorless, toxic fumes when used with high heat. The fumes are known to kill pet birds!

Solution: See Chapter 9

6. **Do you or your children drink from plastic bottles that leach BPA?**

☐ Yes   ☐ No   ☐ Don't know

Hint: Not all plastics are equal. Check the bottom of your bottles for the recycling number.

Problem: Hard polycarbonate (#7 recycling number) bottles may leach an artificial estrogen known as bisphenol A. This chemical is linked to increased risk of miscarriage and birth defects, as well as prostate cancer. Scratches in the plastic, harsh detergents, and boiling liquids exacerbate the leaching.

Solution: See Chapter 4

7. **Do you store your food in plastic?**

☐ Yes   ☐ No   ☐ Don't know

Hint: Tupperware and other storage containers are commonly made with polycarbonate plastic or polyvinyl chloride.

Problem: Plastic containers leach toxic chemicals into the food they store. The dangers increase when food is heated in these plastic containers, since the heat breaks down the plastic and destabilizes it, thus increasing the release of toxic chemicals into your food.

Solution: See Chapter 4

The Bathroom:

8. **Do you use artificially scented household products, including those for skin and hair?**

☐ Yes   ☐ No   ☐ Don't know

Hint: You may suffer from chronic headaches or hives, and be completely unaware of the connection to your perfume or favorite detergent's aroma.

Problem: Almost all of the ingredients used to create fragrances today are made with synthetic compounds that are known toxins and sensitizers.

Solution: See Chapter 5

9. **Look at the labels on your makeup and body care products (get a magnifying glass if necessary!). Do you see words like parabens (including the forms methyl, propyl, or butyl)?**

☐ Yes ☐ No ☐ Don't know

Hint: Parabens are used as preservatives in most cosmetics and personal care products.

Problem: Parabens are dangerous; they have been found in most breast tumors and can be damaging to the immune system.

Solution: See Chapter 5

10. **Does your bathroom contain vinyl wallpaper?**

☐ Yes ☐ No ☐ Don't know

Hint: If it's washable, it is probably made of vinyl.

Problem: PVC (vinyl) is considered to be so toxic that it is banned in some parts of Europe. If you use vinyl wallpaper in high-moisture areas in your home, like the bathroom, it can create a vapor barrier that traps moisture in the wall and encourages mold growth.

Solution: See Chapter 8

11. **Do you use air fresheners?**

☐ Yes ☐ No ☐ Don't know

Hint: Even air fresheners marketed as "all-natural" or "unscented" can contain hazardous chemicals.

Problem: Most air fresheners contain phthalates, chemicals that can cause hormonal abnormalities, birth defects and reproductive problems. In addition to phthalates, air fresheners may contain allergens, volatile organic compounds (VOCs), and cancer-causing chemicals such as benzene and formaldehyde.

Solution: See Chapter 9

The Bedroom, Nursery, or Kid's Room:

12. Is your mattress made of synthetic materials?

☐ Yes   ☐ No   ☐ Don't know

Hint: If you, your spouse, or your child has trouble falling asleep or wakes up often during the night, it could be the fault of your mattress.

Problem: The typical mattress contains chemicals such as polyurethane, Styrofoam, polyester, fire retardants, adhesives, and bonding agents that are recognized carcinogens. These trap the moisture our bodies release during sleep, and this attracts dust mites, which are allergens.

Solution: See Chapter 7

13. Have you purchased cotton-blend or polyester sheets from a regular retail store?

☐ Yes   ☐ No   ☐ Don't know

Hint: Most sheets sold in retail stores are treated with a toxic finish made from formaldehyde that prevents wrinkles and stains. They are labeled as "wrinkle-resistant," "easy care," or "permanent press."

Problem: Formaldehyde, according to the International Agency for Research on Cancer, is a toxic, cancer-causing substance.

Solution: See Chapter 7

14. Do you, your spouse, or your child wear synthetic fabrics and/or sleep in synthetic pajamas?

☐ Yes   ☐ No   ☐ Don't know

Hint: Most synthetic fabrics are treated with chemicals during and after processing, and most children's pajamas are made with fabric that is treated with flame-retardant chemicals, and emit formaldehyde gas.

Problem: Perfluorinated chemicals (PFCs), which include Teflon, are being added to clothing because it makes them last longer and also can make them wrinkle-free. Most clothing labeled "no-iron" contains PFCs. The EPA asserts that PFCs cause cancer.

Solution: See Chapter 7

The Living Room, Den, and Home Office:

15. **Did you recently install new synthetic carpeting?**

☐ Yes   ☐ No   ☐ Don't know

Hint: If you, your spouse or your children have asthma, skin rashes, or food allergies, the condition could be the result of breathing the off-gases from your new carpeting.

Problem: Carpeting is usually made of synthetic fibers that have been treated with pesticides and fungicide. These chemicals are emitted as "off-gas" from new carpeting.

Solution: See Chapter 8

16. **Was the room painted or wallpapered within the last year?**

☐ Yes   ☐ No   ☐ Don't know

Hint: If you smell a strong odor coming from your walls, it's caused by airborne chemicals known as volatile organic compounds, or VOCs. These include ethers (PBDEs) and phthalates, as well as glues or adhesives used in the wallpaper.

Problem: Most VOCs are known to cause serious health problems.

Solution: See Chapter 8

17. **Is your furniture made of particle board?**

☐ Yes   ☐ No   ☐ Don't know

Hint: Particle board is used in shelving and cabinets.

Problem: In most homes, particle board is a major source of formaldehyde in the environment.

Solution: See Chapter 8

18. **Was the furniture's upholstery treated with a flame retardant?**

☐ Yes   ☐ No   ☐ Don't know

Hint: Chances are if you bought your furniture from a department store or conventional furniture store, flame retardants were used to treat the fabric.

Problem: Flame retardants are shown to accumulate in breast milk and negatively affect children's brain function.

Solution: See Chapter 8

Household Cleaners:

19. **Do any of your household cleaners contain ingredients such as ammonia, chlorine bleach, phosphates, or formaldehyde?**

    ☐ Yes   ☐ No   ☐ Don't know

    Hint: If you see a skull and cross bones on the bottle, you can be sure these ingredients are present! If there's a warning on the label that the product is poisonous, dangerous, or flammable, then it's toxic for you to use.

    Problem: Most all-purpose cleaners, ammonia-based cleaners, bleach, metal polish, disinfectants, drain cleaners, glass cleaners, dishwashing detergents, oven cleaners, carpet cleaners, mothballs, mold and mildew cleaners, and scouring powders contain irritants and dangerous chemicals.

    Solution: See Chapter 9

Away from Home:

20. **Do you know what type of cooking oil is used when you are eating at restaurants, cafeterias, and hotels, or on planes?**

    ☐ Yes   ☐ No   ☐ Don't know

    Hint: Most restaurants serve food cooked with partially hydrogenated vegetable oil that contain trans fats.

    Problem: Partially hydrogenated vegetable oil is a toxic substance, harmful in even tiny quantities.

    Solution: See Chapter 10

Scoring This Quiz

- If you checked "yes" for 15 or more questions, you are at "high risk" for exposure to toxic chemicals and should take immediate action to make healthier choices.

- If you checked "yes" for 8 to 14 questions, you are at "moderate risk" but still should take an active approach to making a change toward a greener existence.

- If you checked "yes" to 0 to 7 questions, you're doing great! You might want to consider making one change per month to get you to have a truly super natural home for you and your family!

Take a look at your self-inventory score and think about the choices you make each day, keeping in mind that all of the problems in the quiz have simple, practical solutions to them. Consider the possible cumulative effects on your health and the health of your loved ones. Each choice has a profound impact on your well-being. For self-reflection and to further your understanding, ask yourself:

- Are your choices informed?
- Are they influenced by popular trends, budget, or convenience?
- Why did you choose each product? (Hint: Because you saw them in an ad on TV? Because you grew up using these products?)
- Do you prefer certain brand-name products? Why?
- Does beautiful packaging make you overlook ingredients on the label?

We unwittingly choose products when we are unaware of the health implications or have incomplete information, or when we are led by fads or convenience. But ultimately we pay a big price. Luckily, you can reward yourself the gift of health and vitality by the decisions you make daily. With the guidance I will provide on the following pages, you can make a choice to live a more conscious life that benefits you, your family, and the planet.

What Goes
in You

How to Eliminate Exposure
to Toxic Chemicals in Your
Food and Drinking Water

*"I know a man who gave up smoking, drinking, sex, and rich
food. He was healthy right up to the day he killed himself."*

—JOHNNY CARSON

WHEN MY FRIEND RACHEL TURNED 50, she had plastic surgery on her eyes to remove some of the droopiness and wrinkles that had accumulated over the years. Six weeks after her procedure, there was still lots of bruising, puffiness, and redness around her eyes. "I look like a monster," she said on the phone. She was crying. "I'm not ready to see people until I look better. I'm doing everything my doctor told me to do—I use ice packs and take anti-inflammatory medication, but nothing is helping."

Two weeks later we met for lunch. Rachel wore sunglasses to conceal her eyes. The skin on her face looked pale and puffy. She removed her glasses and I saw dark red lines where the incisions had been made on her lids. The skin on the sides of her eyes was purple and puckered. "I'm back at work now, but I wear tons of makeup," she said, biting into a sugary pastry. "I think my doctor botched the surgery," she added, as she tore open a packet of Equal and started pouring it into her iced tea.

"Wait, don't eat that!" I said, instinctively grabbing her hand to stop the flow of white powder into her glass. "It has bad chemicals in it." I had recently read that Equal contains aspartame, which was shown to cause cancer in animals. "Why do they sell it if it's not safe?" asked Rachel. "They sell cigarettes, don't they?" I countered.

Then it dawned on me: Rachel's skin may not have been healing from the trauma of surgery as quickly as she'd hoped because her body was working overtime to deal with what she'd been eating and drinking. "Do you eat processed food?" I asked. "No," she said, "I don't *think* so. Let's see, for breakfast I usually have dried cereal or white toast with margarine; this morning I had a toaster waffle with lite syrup." "Stop right there!" I shouted. "All those are processed! And I'm sure the syrup wasn't pure maple syrup, was it?" "No," she said. "Then for lunch I usually have a sandwich of some type of lunch meat, and for dessert I have things like diet pudding. Isn't that OK? I'm trying to lose 10 pounds." Rachel continued to tell me what she ate and drank on a regular basis, much of which came out of a box or had added chemicals such as preservatives, artificial colors, and flavor enhancers. I suggested she try something revolutionary: to eat foods that had no label! Or if there was a label—on a yogurt container, for example—it could have no more than five ingredients (a label with a short list is a good thing except when two of five ingredients happen to be sugar!) and she could pronounce every one of them. "I could do that!" she exclaimed with a big smile. She promised she would try this for the next 10 days if I really thought it would help her eyes look better.

Two weeks later she called me. "I'm doing what you told me and my eyes look fantastic!" she squealed. "The redness and puffiness are gone and so is the puckered skin! I guess my plastic surgeon wasn't to blame after all. My body just wasn't healing very quickly." Rachel told me that the "diet" was easier that she thought, even when she was on the road for business. She ate nothing processed, shopped at her local farmer's market, and bought only fresh, whole foods. She ate lots of fresh fruit as well as some squares of organic pure dark chocolate for a treat to substitute for the sweet snacks she was so used to eating.

Now, before you slam this book shut and say "I can't do this! It's not realistic for me to live without foods that have labels!" please consider this: *Your kitchen is one of the most important places in your home to control your exposure to toxic chemicals.* (The other is your bedroom.) Start by making better decisions at the grocery store. But, you may be thinking, there's so much I have to think about when I shop for food! Which fish is OK to eat? Should I check every label for GMO or hidden MSG? Should I not buy an organic avocado if it was flown in from another country? Do I really have to get eggs that were laid by free and happy hens and eat meat from cows that grazed only on grass?

The answer to these questions is no . . . *not all the time!* Don't worry and get stressed out about all the decisions you have to make. You'll then get anxious and fearful or sad and depressed—or worse, angry. I know . . . I've been there. I would avoid going to cocktail parties, or I'd eat at home first, just to avoid the bad food I knew would be served. I would get mad every time I saw a chef on the Food Network cooking with highly processed food, or get stressed when a talk show host oohed and aahed over a dessert made with unnatural ingredients. Then I noticed I was starting to feel self-righteous and smug about the wholesome choices I was making. You don't want to alienate those around you by criticizing their eating habits (even if it is behind their backs!). Friends will be afraid to invite you to their homes for dinner. Or they'll ask you, "What are you *not* eating *now*?"

What I've found works for me is following the 80-20 rule. I try to eat well about 80 percent of the time; the rest of the time I give myself permission to indulge. Recently, my husband and I celebrated our wedding anniversary by traveling to Napa Valley in northern California and having dinner at Ad Hoc restaurant. Its owner, Thomas Keller, is chef of the world-renowned French Laundry. We knew little about the place other than it served organic, local food and was one of the top 100 restaurants in the Bay Area.

The menu arrived—a sheet of paper with only one option: fried chicken, mashed potatoes, salad with bacon, cheese; and, for dessert, chocolate cake with whipped cream. We looked at each other for a moment and then in unison nodded our heads: Yes, let's do it! I haven't indulged like that in over 5 years, and I will admit that it was one of the most delicious meals I've ever had. I enjoyed every bite, and still think about how delicious and decadent that meal was. Will I eat that way every day? No way.

"What we humans consume for food has undergone more profound change in the past century than in the previous one hundred thousand years, yet genetically we have the same bodies and nutritional needs as our hunter-gatherer ancestors. That discrepancy between who we are and what we put into our bodies has sown the seeds for our current epidemics of illness and disease."

—RANDALL FITZGERALD, author of The Hundred Year Lie

I do, however, always make an effort to eat real food, not "foodlike products" as Michael Pollan, author of In Defense of Food, calls food that has been highly processed. Pollan recommends that we "simply avoid any food that has been processed to such an extent that it is more a product of industry than of nature." Margarine is a good example of a foodlike product. Remember, processed food is food processed with chemicals!

To give me peace of mind, I buy the best-quality food I can, even if that means spending $13 a pound for raw, organic almonds. If your concern is that eating healthy is too expensive, consider the words of Alice Waters, natural food pioneer and chef/owner of Chez Panisse in Berkeley, California: "Why wouldn't you want to spend most of your money on food? Food is nourishment and good health. It is the most important thing in life, really."

I agree. Besides, you will be surprised by what you can find at places like Costco, Walmart, and your everyday grocery store that's economical and incredibly good for you. Major chain stores are offering 100 percent organic and natural products to meet the growing demand.

Making slight shifts in what you choose to buy, eat, and drink won't be that difficult. In fact, I'm confident that you'll grow to love the healthy alternatives to processed, manufactured foods. And some of these shifts, if you are diligent with them, can be life-changing beyond the toxin factor. I know one woman who called herself the "Blue Packet Junkie" because she admittedly was addicted to Equal and diet soda for years. She bought Equal packets by the box and diet soda by the case. One day, she decided to eliminate artificial sugar from her diet completely and see what happened. The results were unexpected. Unwanted weight she'd been struggling to lose—those "last 10 pounds"— melted off, and her chronic craving for super-sweet, fatty foods vanished. That was nearly 10 years ago and she's never looked back.

Ready to get started? Here's something you can easily do that won't be radically different from the way you're eating and drinking now. It's avoiding what I call "The Fearsome 5," (which I cover in Chapters 1–4). These are five substances that will zap your energy and vitality, make you look old before your time, and could even make you sick. If you stop consuming these five things, you and your family will be well on your way to better health.

The "Fearsome 5" Things to Avoid

1. Pesticides
2. Food additives: MSG, trans fats (hydrogenated oils), artificial sweeteners
3. Factory-farmed foods
4. Genetically modified foods
5. Unfiltered tap water

For some of these, knowing what to avoid is as simple as reading the ingredient label. Others may require steering clear of an entire category—like diet soda, which contains artificial sweeteners.

Now, turn to chapter 1 to learn about how pesticides affect your health and three ways to make a shift to eating a more healthful diet.

Chapter 1

HOW TO ELIMINATE PESTICIDES AND FIND YOUR FARMER

"Most large grocery chains these days post a sign in at least one section of their stores describing it as a 'health food' section, which has prompted some of us to wonder whether the rest of the supermarket should have signs identifying aisles as filled with 'illness food,' or 'unhealthy food,'. . ."

—RANDALL FITZGERALD, AUTHOR OF
The Hundred-Year Lie

THE TEENAGE DAUGHTER of a friend of mine was babysitting for my child for the first time. Before I left the house, I told her to please feel free to help herself to any food she wanted in my refrigerator or pantry. The next day I touched base with her mom, who said all went well, except that her daughter had phoned her from my home and exclaimed: "Mom, everything in their kitchen is organic. It's so weird!" I was stunned that a 16-year-old would find a kitchen filled with healthy, organic food to be weird, until I realized that "weird" to a teenager usually means something they haven't seen before or been told about.

I would have liked to say to her, imagine picking a fruit or vegetable from your garden, spraying it with bug spray, and then eating it. Now *that* seems weird, doesn't it? Well, that's exactly what we do each day with store-bought nonorganic produce even if we wash it. The term *organic* refers to food that is grown without pesticides, synthetic nitrogen fertilizers, fungicides, or herbicides. Organic foods are minimally processed, with no artificial ingredients, preservatives, or irradiation. And they taste better! Produce is sent to market as close to harvest as possible and may have suffered less nutritional loss by the time you eat it.

Because the chemicals in pesticides are invisible, odorless, and tasteless, the only way to know for sure that a food was grown without pesticides is to buy organic. Even if something *looks* OK, it may not be so healthy for you to eat. For example, don't be fooled by those juicy nonorganic strawberries displayed in the market. They may look luscious, but they have a dark side. Their red color has been enhanced by a fungicide, and they have been infused with methyl bromide, a gas that is injected by tractor into their growing soil. These substances then become part of the fruits' flesh, and can't be washed off. I'm always disturbed when I see a mother feeding a young child a nonorganic strawberry from the case at a natural foods market. She's assuming, as I used to, that if a fruit or vegetable is sold at a store like that it will be pesticide-free. Don't make that assumption. It's always best to read the signs before popping anything into your child's mouth, or your own.

Keep in mind that most fruits and vegetables that are imported from other countries have been treated with chemicals. Much of the garlic used in the United States, for example, comes from China, where chemicals such as growth inhibitors are used to stop the garlic from sprouting. I was startled to find out that garlic from China is often whitened with chlorine to make it look more attractive to consumers. After all, who doesn't pick the whitest garlic bulb in the bunch?

ORGANIC IS BETTER FOOD

Organic foods also have a higher nutritional value, which is important for growing children as well as adults. An organically grown apple can have as much as 300 percent more vitamin C and 61 percent greater calcium content than a conventional or nonorganic apple. The amount of calcium in organic spinach is seven times greater than in nonorganic spinach, and the potassium is an astounding 117 times greater in the organic. In addition, Alyson Mitchell, PhD, food chemist and associate professor who led a

A reminder for pregnant women: Pesticides can cross the placenta and go to the fetus! If you're pregnant, buy as much organic produce as possible.

10-year research study at the University of California, Davis, found that organic tomatoes have as much as 97 percent more cancer-fighting antioxidants as conventionally grown tomatoes.

Given all these facts, why do farmers still use pesticides? Well, mostly it's because they believe it will save more crops from insects, weeds, and disease. But that's not true. Before the 1950s, farmers lost about one-third of their crops each year. Today, even with over 21,000 pesticide products to choose from and pesticide costs exceeding $4 billion a year, farmers still lose one-third of their crops!

"The science might still be sketchy, but common sense tells me organic is better food—better, anyway, than the kind grown with organophosphates, with antibiotics and growth hormones, with cadmium and lead and arsenic (the EPA permits the use of toxic waste in fertilizers), with sewage sludge and animal feed made from ground-up bits of other animals as well as their own manure."

—MICHAEL POLLAN, author of *The Omnivore's Dilemma*

Some nutrition experts say that most of any chemical residue on a nonorganic piece of fruit can be peeled away with its skin. But this sidesteps another important issue: "Pesticides sprayed on our fields poison one in seven farm workers every year, and 800 to 1,000 farmers and farm workers die annually from pesticide exposure," says Anna Lappé, food activist and best-selling author of *Grub: Ideas for an Urban Organic Kitchen.* "By peeling away a pesticide-laden skin, we may be protecting ourselves, but we are failing to protect those who provide us with our food."

WHAT YOU SHOULD KNOW

- Pesticides are toxic to us and the environment.
- A 1997 study from Mount Sinai Medical Center in New York City found that women with high levels of DDE (a derivative of DDT) in their blood were four times as likely to develop breast cancer as women with low levels.
- Pesticides are known to harm the human neurologic system as well as deplete the Earth's protective ozone layer, which can lead to skin cancer.
- Nonorganic peanuts, potatoes (even after they're peeled), and coffee have the largest concentration of pesticides of any food.

3 WAYS TO MAKE A SHIFT

1. Eat organic whenever possible.
2. Find your own farmer.
3. Join a CSA (community-supported agriculture) farm or plant your own garden.

Eat Organic Whenever Possible

Here is a list of a dozen fruits and vegetables that most likely contain pesticide residues. Be sure and choose organic before you eat any of these:

12 Fruits and Vegetables to Buy Organic

Peaches	Grapes	Sweet bell peppers
Apples	Strawberries	Potatoes
Pears	Raspberries	Tomatoes
Green beans	Spinach	Cantaloupe

This list is based on studies by the Consumers Union (CU) and the Environmental Working Group (EWG), which analyzed the amounts and toxicity of pesticide residues found in conventionally grown food samples by the USDA and the FDA. While most of these foods don't exceed safety limits for a dose of a single pesticide, most contain multiple pesticide residues. For example, the FDA detected 30 different pesticides on strawberries they sampled; apples had

Take Your Own Organic Popcorn to the Movies!

Conventional, nonorganic popcorn was ranked as one of the top 10 foods most contaminated with pesticides and chemicals in the FDA's 2003 Total Diet Study.

Also, the Popcorn Board's *2008 Agri Chemical Handbook* lists 33 insecticides, 38 herbicides, five fumigants, 15 fungicides, and four "miscellaneous" chemicals that are approved for use in nonorganic popcorn.

50 different kinds of pesticides. The CU and EWG say that children are most at risk when eating produce that has combined exposures. The Environmental Protection Agency says pesticides block the body's uptake of nutrients critical for proper growth and wreak havoc on development by permanently altering the way a child's system functions. It's been reported that 1-year-olds eat three times as many fresh peaches, per pound of body weight, as do adults, and more than four times as many apples and pears.

10 Nonorganic Fruits and Vegetables with the Fewest Traces of Pesticides

Onions	Cabbage	Bananas
Frozen peas	Avocados	Pineapples
Frozen corn	Mangoes	
Asparagus	Kiwis	

Wash nonorganic produce well. Try using a product called Veggie Wash. It is 100 percent natural and uses ingredients from corn, coconut, and citrus to remove wax, pesticides, soil, toxins, and fingerprints. Be sure to wash organic produce, too. Even though they may be relatively low in pesticides, they can grow near conventionally farmed produce and become exposed through "second-hand" spraying.

Biodynamic: Going beyond Organic

A farming practice that takes organic a step further is called biodynamic. It is based on the work of Austrian philosopher Rudolf Steiner, founder of the Waldorf schools. It looks at a farm as a self-sustaining organism, with the soil, plants, animals, and even the cosmos all interconnected. Like organic farmers, biodynamic growers don't use pesticides or chemical fertilizers. They plant, prune, and harvest according to celestial activity and the Earth's natural rhythms.

Biodynamic produce is said to be the healthiest we can eat. A 1993 study of 16 biodynamic farms in New Zealand showed that the soil quality was much higher—meaning it was richer in minerals and micronutrients—than the soil at their conventional counterparts.

Make Your Own Veggie Wash

Mix ¼ cup vinegar and 2 tablespoons salt into a dish pan filled with filtered water. Soak produce for 15 minutes. Rinse under running water to remove any residue. Enjoy!

You can find biodynamic produce through CSAs and farmers' markets. There are also biodynamic wines on the market (see page 14).

FIND YOUR FARMER

One great way to find fruits and vegetables that are less likely to be treated with pesticides is to find your own farmer. Most of us have our own doctor, dentist, and lawyer—so why not a farmer? Food grown halfway around the world was shipped here by plane, boat, truck, or rail, and no matter which method of transportation it took, lots of petroleum was used and greenhouse gases were emitted along the way. If you're health-conscious as well as ecologically minded, you may want to venture out and find your local farmer. *Business Week* magazine said the local farmer is emerging as a new celebrity. Why not become part of this important movement? Go to your local farmers' market and talk to the farmers directly. Ask if they use pesticides or synthetic fertilizers. Most are an interesting, committed bunch of people. Or better yet, head directly to a farm near you.

Granted, if you happen to live in an area of the country where farmers' markets are just not the norm (although they are growing coast to coast so give

Organic Facts

- If organic farming methods were practiced on the entire planet's food-growing land, it would be like taking more than 1.5 billion cars off the road.
- You can increase your antioxidant intake by 30 percent by choosing organic.
- The average child in America is exposed to five pesticides daily in food and drinking water.

Source: Rodale Institute

it time), then I recommend that you start with your trusted grocer at your favorite supermarket. See if he or she can give you some leads for learning more about your foods and what could be available to you locally from nearby farmers.

A law known as COOL—short for "country of origin labeling"—requires food producers to label where meat, veggies, and fruit come from. It went into effect in September 2008.

JOIN A CSA

Another way to connect with a farmer is to join a CSA (community-supported agriculture) farm. The idea for CSAs was originally conceived in the 1920s by Austrian philosopher Rudolf Steiner, the same person who originated biodynamic farming. Before the growing season, you buy shares in a farm; then, during the season, you—the "shareholder"—get boxes of fresh vegetables, fruits, and herbs (and sometimes eggs and meat). They are selected by the

Industrial Organic

In his book *The Omnivore's Dilemma*, author Michael Pollan writes, "When I think about organic farming, I think family farm, I think small scale . . . I don't think migrant laborers, combines, thousands of acres of broccoli reaching clear to the horizon. To the eye, these farms look exactly like any other industrial farm."

In fact, most big organic operations are owned and operated by conventional mega-farms. As Pollan observes, "The same farmer who is applying toxic fumigants to sterilize the soil in one field is in the next field applying compost to nurture the soil's natural fertility."

It's important to read labels on all organic food products because chances are they come from an industrial organic farm and might even be imported from another country. For example, on a recent visit to Whole Foods, I happened to check the back of a bag of their 365 brand frozen California Vegetable Medley. In small print appeared the words "Product of China." In addition to the cost of flying these vegetables to the United States, this label raises other issues as well, including misleading labeling and the nature of organic standards and practices in China.

Think Before You Drink

Since I try to use organic products as much as I can, I began to look for organic wines about 3 years ago. The choices were very limited back then, even in Napa and Sonoma, California, which is close to where I live. I spoke to one organic vintner who told me he didn't put the word *organic* on his label because he didn't want to be grouped with other vintners making organic wine at that time. He felt they produced an inferior product.

Organic wineries do not use chemicals; some do not add sulfites to their wines, which can cause an allergic reaction in sensitive people. Sulfites act as a preservative and keep white wines from changing to a golden or brown color. (They are not used as often in red wines.) A conventional vintner told me he thought you couldn't make a good-tasting wine without using sulfites.

I found out that in 1998, California grape farmers used 215 million pounds of chemicals. Reports filed with California's agricultural authorities list 17 "highly poisonous" insecticides, fungicides, and herbicides used in conventional grape production. Luckily, more and more wineries are adopting organic and sustainable farming practices. Know that the organic wine industry is still in its infancy and not all wines labeled "organic" are the same. Some use organically grown grapes and add sulfites, while others are 100% organic with nothing else added. Many wines are biodynamic, wherein the growers promote soil vitality, so the roots are forced to grow down deep. "The deeper the roots go, the more minerals they pick up, giving the wine a certain authenticity and sense of place," says biodynamic winemaker Mike Benziger.

To learn more about the wine you drink, talk to the winemaker or to the farmer and delivered directly to you or to a drop-off point every week. There are now more than 1,500 CSAs in the United States. To find a CSA near you, go to www.localharvest.org or www.csacenter.org.

The challenge of buying at a CSA is that you have to learn to cook creatively with the rhythms of the seasons and not just with a shopping list. For example, in winter there might only be kale, Swiss chard, or collard greens available. And what about that funny-looking gnarly brown ball called celeriac? I had avoided it for years until I discovered that it tastes really great in soup.

proprietor at your local wine store. Ask questions, the way you would at the farmers' market, about how they grow their grapes, where they buy them, and so on. The following is a small sampling of organic and biodynamic wineries:

- Benzinger (Napa Valley, CA)
- Bodegas Iranzo (Spain)
- Bonny Doon (Santa Cruz, CA)
- Bonterra Vineyards (Ukiah, CA)
- CADE, a division of PlumpJack (Napa Valley, CA)
- Casa Barranca (Ojai, CA)
- Coates (Orleans, CA)
- Corda (Bloomfield, CA)
- Coturri (Sonoma, CA)
- Cullen (Australia)
- Emiliana (Chile)
- Frey Vineyards (Mendocino, CA)
- Girasole Vineyards (Mendocino, CA)
- Grgich Hills (Napa, CA)
- Guinness McFadden (Mendocino, CA)
- LaRocca (Forest Ranch, CA)
- Le Vin Vineyards (Mendocino, CA)
- Lolonis (Mendocino, CA)
- Marc Kreydenweiss (France)
- Moon Mountain (Sonoma, CA)
- Old River Road Vintners (Ukiah, CA)
- Quivira Dry Creek Valley (Healdsburg, CA)
- Robert Sinskey (Yountville, CA)
- Santa Julia (Argentina)
- Stellar Organic (Capetown, South Africa)
- Yarden (Israel)

Web Sites to Find Local Food Products

- www.eatwellguide.com: provides an online directory of sustainably raised meat, poultry, dairy, and eggs. This means these foods are raised without exhausting natural resources or causing ecologic damage.
- www.eatwild.com: lists local suppliers for grass-fed meat and dairy products.
- www.heritagefoodsusa.com: sells mail-order "traceable" products from small farms whose labels provide details about how they were produced.

- www.localharvest.org: allows searches for farmers' markets, family farms, and other sources of sustainably grown food in your area, where you can buy produce, grass-fed meats, and many other goodies.

There are more food Web sites and food blog information in the Recommended Resources.

PLANT YOUR OWN GARDEN

If "organic" prices frighten you, or you're tired of paying $1 for a pepper, you might try planting your own garden. Now, I'm lucky enough to live in northern California, where the growing season is relatively long, but I grew up in a New York City suburb and had no experience planting a garden. A few years ago I got some information from my local garden supply store, bought organic soil, seeds for carrots, zucchini, and several herbs, as well as some tomato plants that were already in containers. My daughter really wanted to plant pumpkins, so I bought seeds for those as well.

I'll be honest, this first garden wasn't a big success. The herbs dried out because of a lack of water and attention; the carrots sprouted green tops but were as thin as toothpicks when I harvested them (although quite tasty); and the vines for the pumpkins all but took over the entire garden and started choking the tomato plants and zucchini. I did harvest several wonderful tomatoes and a few zucchini, but had to sacrifice the pumpkin, much to my daughter's dismay. After getting better advice, my next garden was much improved. This year I'm planting kale, chard, lettuce, broccoli, strawberries, squash, tomatoes, miniature watermelons, and herbs. It feels good to know I'm eating something that I've nurtured and grown from the ground up. Besides, store-bought produce doesn't come anywhere close to the flavor of something I've grown in my own garden.

If you'd rather not eat food being imported from China, look at the first three digits of the barcode on packaged goods: 690–695 indicates that the product was made in China.

MORE FOOD FOR THOUGHT

Here's what else you can do to reduce pesticides in your diet:

- Be a vigilant consumer. Look at the list of nonorganic fruits and vegetables with high toxicity levels and *don't buy them*. Remember that pesticides can disrupt the endocrine system and be carcinogenic as well.

Pesticides Are Prevalent in Potatoes and Peanut Butter

Most households keep a stash of potatoes and peanut butter because these two foods are so versatile and have a long shelf life. But they usually don't come pesticide free.

Potatoes: Switching to organic potatoes can have a big impact on your health as well as the planet because commercial potatoes are high in pesticides. A 2006 USDA test found that 81 percent of potatoes tested still contained pesticides after being washed and peeled, and the potato has one of the highest pesticide contents of 43 fruits and vegetables tested, according to the Environmental Working Group.

Peanut butter: More acres in the United States are devoted to growing peanuts than any other fruit, vegetable, or nut, according to the USDA. More than 99 percent of peanut farms use conventional farming methods that include fungicides to treat mold, a common problem in peanut crops. Also, many popular brands of peanut butter contain high-fructose corn syrup and partially hydrogenated vegetable oil—the dreaded trans fat! Look for organic brands at the market or go to the health food store and grind your own. You should see nothing but peanuts and maybe some salt on the ingredient label. Brands I enjoy include Arrowhead Mills, Trader Joe's, and Whole Foods' 365, all containing organic Valencia peanuts with no hydrogenated oils or high-fructose corn syrup.

- Make eating organic produce a habit. Go to your health food market, or buy at local farmers' markets.
- Understand the vocabulary. "Conventional" means pesticides were used; "organic" means 95% of the product contains no pesticides; "100% organic" means none of the product contains pesticides.
- Begin with the foods that you and your family are consuming in the greatest quantities. For kids, consider switching to organic baby food, strawberries, rice, milk, bananas, peanut butter, and apples; for adults, consider switching to organic coffee (see "Choosing Coffee with a Conscience" on page 20).

Your Cup of Tea: 3 Healthy Choices

Tea drinking is an ancient tradition dating back 5,000 years in China and India. Regarded as an aid to good health, tea is an outstanding source of antioxidants called catechins, which researchers are now studying for possible use in the prevention and treatment of a variety of cancers. Most commercially made tea is heavily sprayed with pesticides, so it's important to choose organic.

One Chinese tea, known as puer, has for centuries been considered medicinal. It is said to reduce bad cholesterol, lower triglycerides, prevent arteriosclerosis and strokes, aid in weight loss, and help reduce stress. Green puer is one of the most natural, unprocessed teas in the world.

PurePuer Tea is an American company that sells wonderful varieties of organic green and black puer. It is imported from China and is air dried instead of baked at high temperatures. It is available at www.purepuer.com.

In India, the Tulsi herb has been widely known for its health-promoting properties—for body, mind, and spirit—for over 5,000 years. Tulsi is a principle herb of Ayurveda, India's ancient holistic health system. It is

UNSUNG HERO

Jo Robinson, founder/researcher of www.eatwild.com, is an investigative journalist and *New York Times* best-selling author whose books include *Pasture Perfect*. Jo has spent the last decade researching the many benefits of raising animals on pasture. Her Web site is a great resource for locating safe, natural grass-fed beef, lamb, goat, bison, poultry, pork, dairy, and other wild edibles. It provides comprehensive information about the benefits of raising animals on pasture and links consumers with local suppliers of grass-fed products.

Jo's interest in eating wild grew out of a book she coauthored with Artemis Simopoulos, MD, called *The Omega Diet*, which explores the health benefits of the Mediterranean diet. While researching the book, Jo learned that meat from pasture-raised animals is very similar to meat from wild game and that both promote optimal health.

Starting with this insight, she began an exhaustive search of the scientific literature from the 1960s to the present. To date, she has identified hundreds commonly called "sacred basil" or "holy basil" and is rich in antioxidants. Organic India makes terrific certified organic Tulsi tea blends (www.organicindiausa.com).

In South America, yerba maté (pronounced "yerba mahtay") has been used since ancient times as a tea, and is recommended for its rejuvenating, nutritional, and energizing effects, particularly for mental and physical fatigue. In 2005, researchers at the University of Illinois studied 25 different types of maté and found the tea to contain "higher levels of antioxidants than green tea."

Tulsi, yerba maté, and other organic teas can be found at Whole Foods, Trader Joe's, and Starbucks, as well as online at the following:

- Alter Eco (www.altereco-usa.com)
- Assam Tea Company (www.tfactor.us)
- Choice Organic Teas (www.choiceorganicteas.com)
- Eco Teas (www.ecoteas.com)
- Numi Tea (www.numitea.com)
- SerendipiTea (www.serendipitea.com)
- Upton Tea (www.uptontea.com)

of peer-reviewed studies showing that raising animals on pasture is good for the animals, the environment, farm families, and the health of consumers. She gives talks to ranchers, government agencies, sustainable agricultural groups, and the general public.

Jo's book, *When Your Body Gets the Blues*, extended her interest in natural health to human psychology. Working with Marie-Annette Brown, PhD, RN, from the University of Washington, she developed a clinically proven, all-natural program that boosts women's mood and energy levels and tames their appetite. (The book was featured in an hour-long special on PBS.)

Jo lives on Vashon Island in Washington State. She is developing a test garden that features plants with exceptional nutritional value that are similar to plants growing in the wild. Her next book will combine all that she has learned about pastured animals and unusually nutritious fruits, vegetables, nuts, and grains.

For more information, go to: www.eatwild.com.

Choosing Coffee with a Conscience

Coffee is one of the most chemically treated food crops on the planet. It is heavily sprayed with pesticides and grown with chemical fertilizers, herbicides, and fungicides, all known to cause health problems, including cancer and nervous system and reproductive disorders. In fact, most coffee is imported from countries that use chemicals that are banned in the United States.

Coffee is an $18 billion industry—the most traded commodity in the world, second to oil. It's the most popular beverage worldwide, with over 400 billion cups consumed each year. We Americans drink more coffee than any other nation (350 million cups a day)—the average adult drinks more than three cups a day. You'd be hard pressed to go a mile in most parts of the country without finding access to coffee somewhere. But such a high demand is altering the way commercial coffee is grown.

Traditionally, coffee was grown in the shade of tropical forest canopies. These "shade-grown" coffee plantations provided habitat for over 150 species of birds and other wildlife. Over the past 20 years, however, there has been a shift by the major coffee companies to clear the forests and grow coffee in full sun, with no shade canopy at all. Four of 10 coffee fields in Mexico, Columbia, Central America, and the Caribbean have been converted from shaded plantations to sun-grown plantations. This has had a negative impact on the environment and wildlife. Studies in Colombia and Mexico found 90 percent fewer bird species in sun-grown coffee regions than in shade-grown ones. When the habitats of birds are removed, there are more pests, which then increase the need for pesticides.

Coffee farmers are negatively affected as well. Gourmet coffee that sells for $8 to $9 a pound in the United States pays coffee farmers just 11 to 12 cents a pound. And according to a 1995 report from the World Wide Fund for Nature, in Kenya, for example, coffee harvesting is almost exclusively the domain of women and their children, while male workers spray coffee trees with toxic pesticides 6 to 11 hours a day. Organic farmers who grow coffee on small, shaded, wildlife-friendly, and pesticide-free land often can't compete in the marketplace, and their businesses often fail. They then become unable to pay for food, clothing, their children's education, and health care. That's why eco-conscious companies are making a "fair trade" commitment to support smaller growers.

So what can you do as a consumer? You don't have to give up coffee. There is one very practical action you can take: Look for "shade-grown" on the label. This type of coffee farming uses significantly fewer chemicals than does sun coffee. In addition, shade trees provide natural mulch, which reduces the need for chemical fertilizers. Also choose "organic," which is grown without pesticides and fertilizers, and "Certified Fair Trade," which means that farmers are guaranteed a minimum price for their coffee.

Some coffees are labeled as all three, but if you have a choice, it's best to buy organic, since most organic coffee is shade-grown. Buying organic, fair trade, and shade grown coffee costs a little more, but what you're paying for is a better-tasting, healthier brew . . . as well as peace of mind.

Coffee Choices

Avoid instant and flavored coffees, which contain many chemical additives, and opt for freshly ground coffee beans instead. If you prefer your brew decaffeinated, drink steam- or water-processed varieties to avoid the hexane and methylene chloride used in the decaffeinating process. Use unbleached paper coffee filters, cotton cloth filters, or a French press, which has a fine-mesh filter.

Some good organic, fair trade, and/or shade grown brands of coffee include the following:

- Audubon Premium
- Caffe Ibis
- Caribou Coffee Company
- Counter Culture Coffee
- Equal Exchange
- Green Mountain Coffee Roasters (in partnership with Newman's Own Organic)
- Grounds for Change
- Higher Ground Roasters
- Peace Coffee
- Sacred Grounds Organic Coffee Roasters
- Thanksgiving Coffee Company

Starbucks agreed to double its purchases of certified Fair Trade coffee to 40 million pounds in 2009.

Chapter 2

FORGET FOOD ADDITIVES

Giving Up MSG, Trans Fats, and Artificial Sweeteners

"Eating rice cakes is like chewing on a foam coffee cup, only less filling."

—DAVE BARRY

UNLIKE SALT, spices, and herbs, which have been used for centuries to naturally enhance the flavor of food, most food additives today are made in a high-tech laboratory. They enhance taste, but they do a lot of other things, too—like prevent sliced ham from turning grey, extending shelf life (almost indefinitely), and stimulating your appetite to eat (and buy!) more.

Synthetic food additives grew out of the perfume industry. IFF, International Flavors and Fragrances, not only makes best-selling perfumes for companies such as Estée Lauder, Calvin Klein, Lancôme, and Clinique, and scents found in bath soap, shampoo, furniture polish, and floor wax, it also makes the aromas found in processed foods, such as frozen dinners. It has been estimated that as much as 90 percent of a food's flavor can be attributed to its smell!

At least 100 new synthetic additives are added to the food supply each year, so it's important to read labels. That means not just the expiration (freshness) date! Even though packaged goods have a dizzying amount of information, make a habit of seriously looking at the ingredient list on the label of every product you buy. While most food additives are safe, some haven't been adequately tested, and a few could be dangerous.

Some food additives and colorings cause allergy-like symptoms or are suspected carcinogens. According to the Center for Science in the Public Interest, the additives in the following list are unsafe in the amounts typically consumed by the average American or are very poorly tested and should be avoided. Besides being among the most questionable, they are used primarily in foods of low nutritional value.

1. Acesulfame K: Artificial sweetener found in baked goods, chewing gum, gelatin desserts, and diet soda.

2. Artificial colorings: Blue 1 and 2, Green 3, Red 3, and Yellow 6, found in beverages, candy, and baked goods.

3. Aspartame: Artificial sweetener found in frozen desserts, diet soda, and tabletop sweetener (Equal and NutraSweet).

4. BHA (butylated hydroxyanisole): Antioxidant found in cereals, chewing gum, vegetable oil, and potato chips.

5. Sodium nitrite, sodium nitrate: Preservative, coloring, and flavoring in bacon, ham, frankfurters, luncheon meats, smoked fish, and corned beef.

6. Trans fats (partially hydrogenated vegetable oil): Fat, oil, and shortening found in stick margarine, crackers, fried restaurant foods, baked goods, icing, and microwave popcorn.

For more information about additives to avoid, see the Recommended Resources.

I'm going to cover three of the most common additives here, and help you spot them on food labels. If you can shift away from these, you'll probably be avoiding lots of other additives at the same time. Food additives like to travel in groups, so it's easy to make a tremendous change for the better just by taking note of these three:

1. MSG

2. Trans fats

3. Artificial sweeteners

MSG: IT'S NOT JUST IN CHINESE FOOD

When I was in my twenties, I used to get a headache every time I ate a meal at a Chinese restaurant. When I discovered that the source of

Food Dyes Are Made with Synthetic Chemicals

Artificial colors are made from petroleum as well as coal tar (an extract of coal that the Environmental Protection Agency [EPA] says is highly toxic) and are found in things such as fruit drinks, sports drinks, candy, ice cream, ices, pet food, and store-bought cakes and cookies (think blueberry bagels and green St. Patrick's Day bagels and muffins, too!).

A 2007 study, commissioned by the United Kingdom's Food Standards Agency, found that six artificial colors and one preservative caused hyperactivity and temper tantrums in normal children. Spotting additives is not easy; they are listed in ingredients lists, but the print is often very small. Besides, some foods are sold without any packaging. And additives may be used in restaurant and take-out food. Best bet if you or your child likes brightly colored candy? Go for the organic ones (jelly beans, too!) because they will have natural food coloring.

The Center for Science in the Public Interest is asking the FDA to ban eight artificial food colors used in processed foods in the United States and to require warning notices on the labels of foods that contain them.

my headaches was the MSG (monosodium glutamate) that was added to the food, I began making sure to say "No MSG, please" along with my order. MSG is the most widely used flavor enhancer in the world, yet it has absolutely no nutritional value and—ironically—no flavor of its own. What you may not realize is that aside from showing up abundantly in the food served in places such as Burger King, McDonald's, Wendy's, Taco Bell, TGI Friday's, Chili's, Applebee's, Denny's, and KFC, MSG is also in most processed brand name foods, such as Campbell's soups, Doritos, Lays potato chips, Betty Crocker's Hamburger Helper, Heinz canned gravy, Swanson frozen meals, and Kraft salad dressings. It's also in dried soup mixes, prepared gravy, bullion cubes, and most processed food for children, including canned or packaged spaghetti, microwavable cups, and much more.

In short, it's everywhere most Americans look when it comes to their next convenient meal.

A Little History

For thousands of years kombu (a type of seaweed) was added to foods in Japan to enhance flavor. In 1908 a Japanese scientist discovered that the active ingredient in kombu, glutamate, could be synthesized and added to food to make it more savory. During World War II, Americans noticed that Japanese army rations, unlike their own, tasted delicious. Following the war, MSG, the flavor-enhancing ingredient in the Japanese rations, was introduced to US food manufacturers, and it took off.

While some people can eat MSG with no adverse effects, many have severe, even life-threatening physical and neurologic reactions to it. MSG works by exciting and increasing the sensitivity of your taste buds. In other words, it makes your nervous system believe that the foods you are eating—especially those that are low-fat or nonfat—are tastier than they actually are.

There is increasing scientific evidence that taste cells on the tongue are not the only things that MSG stimulates. According to neurosurgeon Russell Blaylock, MD, author of *Excitotoxins: The Taste That Kills*, when neurons in the brain are exposed to MSG, they become overexcited and fire their impulses rapidly until they reach a state of extreme exhaustion. Several hours later these neurons die, as if the cells were excited to death. That's why Dr. Blaylock calls MSG an "excitotoxin."

Dr. Blaylock believes that MSG can damage children's brains by affecting the development of the nervous system so that years later they may have learning and emotional difficulties (attention-deficit and attention-deficit hyperactivity disorders, autism) or hormonal problems. He also links cumulative exposure of MSG to an accelerated onset of many neurodegenerative diseases, such as Alzheimer's disease, Parkinson's disease, amyotrophic lateral sclerosis (ALS, or Lou Gehrig's disease), and Huntington's disease. John Olney, MD, a leading researcher in the field at Washington University School of Medicine, St. Louis, has estimated that the MSG in a single bowl of commercial soup, drunk with a can of diet, aspartame-sweetened soda, would raise a 2-year-old child's blood level of MSG to six times the concentration demonstrated to cause brain damage in animals.

Animal studies may not always translate to humans, but then again, they might. We just don't know exactly how much of a toxin such as MSG is needed to have an effect on individuals. Every person has a different tolerance level, and you won't know what your threshold is until it may be too late. So why take the risk?

Fat Rats and MSG

Why is MSG in so many of the foods we eat? Is it just to make the food taste better? Or could there be a more subversive reason? According to John Erb, author of *The Slow Poisoning of America*, MSG is added to food because it is addictive and food manufacturers want people to eat more of the food they sell. Erb writes that food companies want to make profits; they are not interested in curing disease or even preventing it. Erb cites hundreds of studies from around the world in which scientists created obese mice and rats to use in diet or diabetes test studies. Since no strain of rat or mice is naturally obese, the scientists made them so by injecting them with MSG when they were first born.

WHAT YOU SHOULD KNOW

- Even if you don't eat processed food or frequent fast-food restaurants, you are probably still consuming MSG because it goes under aliases such as "vegetable protein," "natural flavoring," and "spices." The most common one is "hydrolyzed vegetable protein," used to increase the protein content of a wide variety of foods.

- Some unexpected sources of MSG include restaurant soups, reduced-fat milk, chewing gum, vitamin-enriched foods, candy, cigarettes, medications, mineral supplements, and soy protein.

The good news is that it's actually not difficult to avoid MSG if you know what to look for. Here are some tips.

3 WAYS TO MAKE A SHIFT

1. Minimize fast food and restaurant food, not just Chinese food.
2. Read food labels. MSG is often present in foods that are not labeled as containing MSG but do.
3. Minimize consumption of processed foods. Items in cans, boxes, bags, and frozen foods such as fruits and vegetables can be totally fine, as long as you read the label to make sure there aren't food additives included.

Hidden Sources of MSG*

If you see any of these ingredients on a food label, it's your cue that the food contains MSG:

Glutamic acid	Sodium caseinate
Textured protein	Gelatin
Hydrolyzed protein	Yeast extract
Monopotassium glutamate	Yeast food
Calcium caseinate	Autolyzed yeast

The following ingredients *may* contain MSG, or they may create MSG during processing:

Flavors and flavorings	Carrageenan
Seasonings	Maltodextrin
Natural flavors	Powdered milk
Soy protein isolate	Anything protein fortified
Bouillon	Anything enzyme modified
Malt extract	Anything ultra-pasteurized
Barley malt	

TRANS FATS:
TRASH 'EM—THEY'RE TREACHEROUS

It finally happened—the thing I had been dreading since my daughter started to have play dates away from my watchful eye. She came home from a friend's house and sheepishly announced that she had eaten McDonald's Chicken McNuggets.

"Oh, really," I said nonchalantly, attempting to hide my dismay and disappointment. Even though I raised my daughter on organic produce with little or no processed food, I knew this day would come. At age 8, she ate the dreaded food made from highly processed reconstituted chicken that is battered, breaded and mixed with toxic additives and preservatives, then deep-fried in trans fat-laden, partially hydrogenated oil. "How'd it taste?" I asked, afraid

* Source: Price-Pottenger Foundation

Slow Food Movement

The opposite of fast food is "slow food," where ingredients are selected meticulously, cooked with care, and savored with good company. It's a global, grassroots movement that began in 1989 as a protest against the opening of a McDonald's in Rome. It now has thousands of members around the world who believe that food brings people together, linking the pleasure of food with traditions, farms, plants, animals, and fertile soils. Slow Food USA seeks to inspire and empower Americans to build a food system that is sustainable, healthy, and delicious. For more information, go to www.slowfoodusa.org.

to hear her answer. "OK," she replied. "I only ate two." I was relieved. Then, a few hours later, she had diarrhea. From that day on, she hasn't touched the stuff.

But chicken nuggets are also made in good restaurants where chefs will deep fry chicken parts in partially hydrogenated vegetable oil, leaving them with up to 20 grams of fat—most of which is saturated—per 3-ounce serving. If you're looking for a healthier version, you might try making the recipe on page 32 at home. It's pretty easy, and it tastes a lot better than its deep-fried alternative.

If you can't remember the last time you made a meal from scratch, try preparing some nonprocessed food just once a week. Use butter and olive oil (even coconut oil) in place of margarine, which is high in trans fats. They taste better, and appear to be better for you.

Chances are you are consuming trans fats without even knowing it. Many, possibly most restaurants—even upscale ones—cook their food in partially hydrogenated oil. Why should you care? Because when manufacturers add hydrogen to vegetable oil (a process called hydrogenation), it creates artery-clogging trans fats, and scientists report that trans fats are harmful in even tiny quantities. They can clog

According to the Center for Science in the Public Interest, trans fat is the most harmful fat, and has been causing about 50,000 fatal heart attacks a year.

linings of blood vessels and surfaces in the brain, and they are linked to obesity, heart disease, diabetes, high cholesterol, and even sudden cardiac death.

You might be thinking that you or your kids eat only one or two

MYTH: Coconut oil is a "bad" fat because it is saturated and should be avoided at all costs.

TRUTH: Coconut oil has gotten a bad rap in the last 20 years—for all the wrong reasons. A negative campaign against saturated fats in general led to most food manufacturers' abandoning coconut oil in favor of the polyunsaturated oils that come from the main cash crops in the United States, particularly soy. But studies conducted on traditional tropical populations that consume large amounts of coconut oil show just the opposite. People who have a diet high in coconut oil are healthier and have less heart disease, cancer, and colon problems than people who eat other fats. With a long shelf life and a melting point of 76°F, coconut oil is ideal for cooking and baking.

store-bought cookies at a time, and maybe a few pretzels and a candy or two, so how bad could that be? Well, based on an analysis of data collected from the massive Harvard Nurses Study, a Harvard research group found that consuming just 1 gram of trans fat on a regular, daily basis is likely to increase your risk of heart disease by 20 percent. So let's do the math: The FDA says that any food that contains less than 0.5 gram of trans fat per serving "shall be expressed as zero." That means that if you eat one serving each of cookies, chips, and pretzels, all containing 0.4 gram per serving, you have just consumed 1.2 grams of trans fat, even though each of the labels claim that the products contain 0 grams of trans fat per serving!

Yes, food manufacturers are kind of tricking us by this suspicious math. The fact of the matter is that small quantities of trans fats do add up, just like calories add up after one, two, and three handfuls of potato chips. When it comes to trans fats, the concept of "moderation" doesn't really apply. And like MSG, trans fats are easy to nix from your diet without feeling deprived. It's getting easier, too, as food companies are beginning to phase out the use of trans fats.

One person who helped bring the evils of trans fats to the public eye is Stephen Joseph, founder of BanTransFats.com. He's a lawyer who sued Kraft/Nabisco in 2003 to ban the marketing and sale of trans fat–laden Oreo cookies to children, and to prevent Kraft from continuing to distribute Oreo cookies to young kids in schools. As a result of the lawsuit, Kraft agreed to reduce or eliminate trans fat in all its cookies and crackers.

But, you don't have to threaten a lawsuit to get what you want! At restaurants, bakeries, and other places where you buy food with no Nutrition Facts labels, ask what kind of oil or fat they use. Don't be shy. When you ask, you are sending a message to the seller of the food that you don't want to eat trans fats. And try thinking out of the box . . . literally. My daughter now enjoys eating Nori, Japanese seaweed strips that I buy at a market selling Asian specialty foods. She thinks they're green potato chips and I don't correct her.

WHAT YOU SHOULD KNOW

- The National Academy of Sciences has stated that trans fats raise bad cholesterol and lower good cholesterol. No other food does that.

- Studies have shown that eating trans fats can lead to major increases in cancer, arthritis, fatigue, and many chronic illnesses in all population groups.

- In addition to finding trans fats in fast-food restaurants, be aware that trans fats are being used in the takeout food you order from grocery delis, including fresh-baked supermarket muffins, donuts, breads, tortillas, and cookies.

- Trans fats are hidden in many processed and packaged foods and snacks, including salad dressings, french fries, mayonnaise and other spreads, and most packaged foods, such as chips, pretzels, candies (e.g., Tootsie Rolls and Snickers), and prepared meals.

- Of all processed foods, frozen apple pie, donuts, crackers, and cookies top the list for trans fats, says *Consumer Reports*.

Which Oils Are Best to Use?

The generic term *vegetable oil* refers to a blend of a variety of oils, often including corn and soybean oils (which, if not organic, are most likely genetically modified). Olive oil has no trans fats and is great for salads and cooking. Also try these oils for frying, baking, and grilling. They have a high smoke point, the temperature at which the oil begins to decompose and visible fumes (smoke) are given off.

- Macadamia nut oil
- Rice bran oil
- Grapeseed oil
- Coconut oil
- Hemp seed oil

3 WAYS TO MAKE A SHIFT

1. Become a careful label reader, especially focusing on ingredient lists. If you see "partially hydrogenated" or "shortening," don't eat that food.

2. Choose natural foods—ones with ingredient lists you can understand. Or, better yet, eat whole foods and snacks such as organic raisins, raw nuts, and fresh fruit, with no ingredient list at all.

3. Don't be swayed by advertising. Many prepared foods that are marketed as "convenient" or "kid-friendly" contain trans fats and are poor in nutrition.

Make Your Own Chicken Nuggets

Here's a recipe for homemade chicken nuggets that make a great hors d'oeuvre, or finger food at cocktail parties. Kids love them too!

INGREDIENTS:

    2 lbs. boneless, skinless chicken breasts
    3 tablespoons butter, melted, or olive oil
    2 teaspoons Worcestershire sauce
    ½ cup dried bread crumbs (plain or Italian)
    ⅓ cup grated Parmesan cheese

DIRECTIONS:

Cut chicken into 1-inch pieces. Combine chicken, melted butter or oil, and Worcestershire sauce in a 1-quart freezer bag. Combine the bread crumbs and Parmesan cheese in a second freezer bag. Tape the two bags together. Label and freeze.

To prepare for serving, thaw and remove the chicken pieces from the marinade. Shake them in the bread crumb bag to coat, a few at a time.

Preheat oven to 450. Arrange chicken on a greased cookie sheet. Bake 7–9 minutes or until no longer pink in the center.

PREP TIME: 20–30 MINUTES.
Serves 4

Source: www.chefmom.com

ARTIFICIAL SWEETENERS:
SCARY SWEET STUFF

Like my friend Rachel, whom I mentioned in chapter 1, most people who use artificial sweeteners assume the product was thoroughly tested for safety by the FDA. This is just not true. Reports are regularly being released from independent scientific labs, universities, and research facilities about the health hazards of artificial sweeteners in animals.

You may think these findings don't apply to humans, but scientists are testing rats using dosages that are proportional to the amount a human would ingest during the course of the day. And they are finding that the animals are getting cancerous tumors!

In 2007, a long-term study from an Italian cancer institute revealed that aspartame—a synthetic chemical composed of the amino acids phenylalanine and aspartic acid—increases the occurrence of lymphomas, leukemias, and breast cancer in rats. Aspartame is found in all kinds of sugar-free and "diet" foods and beverages, including sodas, juices, gums, candies, yogurts, puddings, and hundreds of other products that kids and adults consume.

If you want to lose weight and you're thinking that diet soda is a better choice than the sugar-sweetened variety, you'd be wrong. A 2005 study from the University of Texas Health Science Center, San Antonio, shows that diet soft drinks not only don't help weight loss, they actually may contribute to weight *gain* by stimulating appetite and bringing on a craving for carbohydrates—especially the kind high in fat and processed sugar. The American Cancer Society concurs that people who use artificial sweeteners gain more weight than those who avoid them.

Every artificial sweetener on the market uses a different type of chemical molecule to trick the tongue into thinking it is tasting something sweet. Currently, the FDA has approved five artificial sweeteners for use in the United States: saccharin (found in Sweet'N Low and Tab), aspartame (in NutraSweet, Equal, Diet Coke, and Diet Pepsi), sucralose (Splenda; also in Diet Hanson's sodas), neotame (in newer formulations of Tang and some sparkling waters), and acesulfame potassium (Sweet One, Sunnett, and, with Splenda, Diet Snapple and Diet Rite). Others are under review and will come on the market soon.

Is Splenda Really Splendid?

Sucralose was discovered in 1976 by Leslie Hough and Shashikant Phadnis, researchers who were testing chlorinated sugars as chemical substances produced during a reaction. When Hough asked Phadnis to *test* the powder, Phandis took that to mean *taste* it, so he did. He found the compound to be exceptionally sweet. You can imagine how they thought they'd come up with a brand-new sweetener!

They worked on their formula for another year and arrived at something 600 times sweeter than regular table sugar. It took much longer for the formula to find government approval, though; Canada finally allowed it for use as a sweetener in 1991, followed 7 years later by the United States. By then it was being mixed with fillers such as dextrose and maltodextrin (forms of glucose taken from corn) and marketed as Splenda.

Today Splenda is found in products such as candy, breakfast bars, soft drinks, and low-fat or low-sugar ice cream. Restaurants and coffee shops offer the distinctive yellow packets along with sugar, Equal, and Nutra-Sweet. You can also buy Splenda for baking at home. It has overtaken Equal as the number one artificial sweetener on the market.

Because Splenda is marketed as a derivative of real sugar, people think it is a natural product and a better alternative to other artificial sweeteners and sugar (presumably because Splenda lacks the calories). But its marketing can be deceptive. The other day, for example, I attended a fundraiser for breast cancer at which bottles of Nutrisoda (isn't that an oxymoron?) were being handed out to guests. This "nutrient-enhanced soda" in beautifully designed glass bottles had names such as Focus (with B vitamins), Immune (with amino acids), and Radiant (with antioxidants). I took a few sips of one before noticing a strange sensation in my chest. Then I read the small print on the label: It was sweetened with sucralose. It also said "natural fruit flavors" and, in small print, "contains no fruit juice." Instead there were artificial colors and preservatives. And they call this a natural health drink!

A 2005 study published in the *Journal of Head and Face Pain* identified sucralose as a possible trigger for migraine patients. Concerns have been raised about the effect of sucralose on the thymus, an organ that is important to the immune system. Remember this: Splenda is not a natural product. It is not grown or found in nature.

WHAT YOU SHOULD KNOW

- Artificial sweeteners are not limited to diet sodas. They are in sugar-free gums, candies, yogurts, and tons of sugar-free desserts.

- There is a 41% increase in risk of being overweight for every can or bottle of diet soft drink a person consumes each day, according to Sharon P. Fowler, MPH, and colleagues at the University of Texas Health Science Center, San Antonio.

- Aspartame contains methanol, which the body breaks down into formaldehyde—the same substance used in the embalming process. In a living person it can cause cancer, according to the International Agency for Research on Cancer. According to Dr. Blaylock, "Drinking even one diet cola a day can cause formaldehyde buildup in cells, so that the amount of the toxin increases daily."

3 WAYS TO MAKE A SHIFT

1. Use agave nectar. Produced in Mexico from several species of cactus, agave nectar is a syrup-like liquid, a little thinner than honey. It dissolves easily in cold liquids and can be used as a sugar substitute in baking (use ⅓ cup agave syrup for every 1 cup of sugar in the original recipe). Because it has a negligible effect on blood sugar, it may be safe for those with diabetes.

Some of the Many Uses of Honey

With its antiseptic, antibiotic, antifungal, and antibacterial properties, honey is more than just an alternative to artificial sweeteners.

- Apply to skin to treat rashes and abrasions and to moisturize.

- Use it as an antibacterial "soap" for facial blemishes and acne caused by cosmetics or allergies.

- Dab onto canker sores, blisters, and mouth ulcers to promote healing.

Honey also makes an excellent natural preservative. Unprocessed honey found in ancient tombs was determined to still be edible. It never spoils!

2. Consider stevia. Stevia is a noncaloric herb, native to Paraguay. It's been used as a sweetener for centuries. Stevia comes in liquid as well as powder form and is 300 times sweeter than sugar. It also is diabetes-friendly. Before buying a large quantity of stevia, give it a taste test; the flavor is too strong for some, and it may not suit your fancy.

3. Try honey that is produced by bees from the nectar of flowers. Raw honey is best—it comes straight from the hive and is not heated, which can kill health-enhancing enzymes. Honey has been used since ancient times as a food and as a medicine. It can be used to treat burns, may help with allergies, and has been shown to be an antioxidant. Manuka honey (from New Zealand) is considered to be top of the line in terms of health benefits.

UNSUNG HERO

Weston A. Price is almost unknown to today's medical community and to most people. Weston was a dentist whose 1939 book *Nutritional and Physical Degeneration* describes the fieldwork he did in the 1920s and 1930s among

More Alternative Sweeteners

Besides white sugar (which is sprayed with pesticides, processed, and chemically bleached) and artificial sweeteners, try the following:

- Raw or unprocessed sugar called muscovado, also known as rapadura. This type of sugar still contains the minerals and vitamins from the sugar cane plant that refined white sugar doesn't.

- Blackstrap molasses, which is rich in minerals.

- Maple syrup (grade B is the least processed type and is richer in minerals than grade A).

- Date sugar, made by dehydrating dates and grinding them into a granulated sugar.

- Fig syrup, made by boiling figs in water (similar to molasses in consistency).

- Barley malt and brown rice syrup, considered to be the healthiest sweeteners in the natural-foods industry.

MYTH: Diet soda is better than regular because it has fewer, if any, calories from sugar.

TRUTH: While the sugar content of soda is a major factor contributing to obesity and dental problems, a bigger health concern is the phosphoric acid content. When you consume phosphoric acid, it increases phosphorus levels in your body, which may deplete calcium, thus elevating your risk of osteoporosis. This is in addition to concerns about the artificial sweeteners in diet soda.

various world cultures. He has been called the "Charles Darwin of Nutrition." In his search for the causes of dental decay and physical degeneration that he observed in his dental practice, he studied isolated nonindustrialized populations, such as Eskimos, Australian aborigines, New Zealand Maori, and the Indians of South America. He found that these native people had beautiful straight teeth free from decay, as well as strong bodies.

When Weston analyzed the diets of these isolated primitive peoples, he found that they were filled with nutrient-dense whole foods. These diets provided at least four times the amounts of water-soluble vitamins and calcium and other minerals, plus at least 10 times the amounts of fat-soluble vitamins (A and D), from animal foods such as fish, eggs, shellfish, organ meats, and butter made from the milk of cows eating green grass.

Weston also discovered another fat-soluble vitamin that he called Activator X; others refer to it as the Price Factor or X Factor. It's now believed to be vitamin K2, a powerful catalyst that—like vitamins A and D—helps the body absorb and utilize minerals. It was present in the diets of all the healthy population groups he studied, but unfortunately, has almost completely disappeared from the modern western diet.

Beyond their nutrient density, all of the diets of the traditional people whom Weston studied shared the following characteristics:

- They used no refined or denatured foods.
- They contained animal products.
- They provided some raw animal foods.
- The foods were high in enzymes.

Pause before Sipping Soda

In response to consumer pressure, the FDA is beginning to analyze soft drinks for benzene. Of the over 100 soft drinks and other beverages they've tested so far, five contained levels of benzene (a cancer-causing chemical linked to leukemia) that exceed federal standards set for drinking water. While the FDA's benzene limit for drinking water is 5 parts per billion (ppb), researchers found levels as high as 79 ppb in the drinks, with most having at least some detectable level of benzene present. If you see the words "sodium benzoate" or "potassium benzoate" on the label, it means there's benzene present in the form of a preservative.

Researchers from the University of Minnesota surveyed children age 8 to 13 about their soft drink habits. They discovered that parents were the role models for their kids' eating habits, even more so than their peers. So the next time you want to pop open a can of soda, pause for a moment. One of the best things you could do is drink a glass of water instead.

Here's something else to think about: The nine teaspoons of sugar contained in just one can of regular soda supply 180 calories, almost 10 percent of the daily calorie requirement for an average adult. If you cut out the soda, you effectively cut out the calories and can see the weight drop off automatically *even if you do nothing else.*

Five Soft Drinks That Contain Excessive Benzene Levels

- Safeway Select Diet Orange
- Crush Pineapple

- Seeds, grains, and legumes were soaked, fermented, or naturally leavened.
- Animal bones were used to make broth.
- Total fat content varied from 30% to 80% of calories, with only 4% coming from polyunsaturates.
- The diets provided nearly equal amounts of omega-6 and omega-3 fatty acids.
- All the diets contained some salt.

The Weston A. Price Foundation is a nonprofit organization dedicated to promoting the ideas of the late Dr. Price—in particular, the restoration of nutrient-dense foods to the human diet—through education, research, and

- AquaCal Strawberry Flavored Water Beverage
- Crystal Light Sunrise Classic Orange
- Giant Light Cranberry Juice Cocktail

Source: FDA

Alternatives to Soda

- A new natural, sugar-free diet soda hit the market in 2008. Called Zevia, it is sweetened with stevia, an herb native to rainforests, and made with natural colorings like annatto, from the seed of the achiote tree. To find a store that sells Zevia, visit www.zevia.com.

- Safeway stores (including Vons, Dominicks, and Randalls) sell LIVE Energy Drinks containing all-natural ingredients with some organic components. LIVE comes in four flavors, and 50% of the profits are donated to global charities.

- If you want to go completely natural, try drinking sparkling water mixed with a dash of fruit juice.

- Try coconut water as a great sports drink alternative. It is rich in potassium and is now sold in many grocery stores. Two good-tasting brands of 100% natural coconut water are O.N.E. and Amy & Brian.

activism. It supports a number of movements that are consistent with its mission, including accurate nutrition instruction, organic and biodynamic farming, pasture-feeding of livestock, community-supported farms, and honest and informative labeling. Specific goals include establishment of universal access to clean, certified raw milk and a ban on the use of soy formula for infants.*

For more information, see www.nourishingourchildren.org and www.westonaprice.org.

* According to the Price Foundation, babies fed soy-based formula have 13,000 to 22,000 times more estrogen compounds in their blood than babies fed milk-based formula. Infants exclusively fed soy formula receive the estrogenic equivalent (based on body weight) of at least five birth control pills per day. Megadoses of estrogen (phytoestrogens) in soy formula have been implicated in the current trend toward increasingly premature sexual development in girls and delayed or retarded sexual development in boys.

Critics Call High-Fructose Corn Syrup a Four-Letter Word

While high-fructose corn syrup (HFCS) isn't considered a synthetic food additive, it is not a "natural" ingredient, either. In fact, it's a substance you might consider avoiding if you want to remain healthy. HFCS is almost certainly made from genetically modified corn, and genetically modified enzymes are used to process it. (See chapter 3 for more information on genetically modified foods.)

HFCS is ubiquitous today, found in so many products, including soft drinks and processed foods too numerous to name. One surprising place is in most popular nonfat yogurts. If you check the labels you'll surely find high-fructose corn syrup as #2 on the list, followed by modified corn starch and artificial sugar. And you thought you were eating a low-fat, healthy food!

Chapter 3

FORGO FACTORY FARMS, FEEDLOTS, AND "FRANKENFOODS"

"We are living in a world today where lemonade is made from artificial flavors and furniture polish is made from real lemons."

—Alfred E. Neuman

IT'S INCREDIBLE TO THINK how far we've come in the transportation of foods from around the world. You can be sitting in a fine restaurant in New York City eating wild salmon caught in Alaska; the avocado in your salad could have been plucked from a Chilean tree; and the organic raspberries in your dessert could have been harvested in California. But with the technology that brings fresh foods from afar come advancements in generating foods in massive quantities that lose their ties to Mother Nature.

You're more likely to find farmed fish, genetically modified crops, and beef, poultry, or eggs that have some rather unnatural beginnings in restaurants as well as at your local supermarket. For this very reason, I prefer to shop at my local farmer's market, where I know the origins of my foods and that they have not been shipped thousands of miles and exposed to who-knows-what along the way.

I enjoy shopping at my farmer's market almost as much as I enjoy visiting a good art gallery. They both give me a sense of awe and wonder—the way things are arranged, the colors, the shapes, all melding together like a giant painting, delighting my senses. Each booth at the market is like its own work of art, but this art is touchable and affordable and you get to take it home with you.

Feeling entranced, I sometimes stroll around the market in a dreamy state while I revel in the bounty that is on display. I'm usually snapped out of my reverie by my husband, who inevitably shows up carrying at least two bags brimming with all sorts of green leafy things and points out that I have nothing in my bag other than a box of ripe strawberries, a fragrant bunch of lavender, or a jar of local honey. Fortifying myself with a cup of organic coffee and a few nibbles from an artisan cheese vendor, I head over to the local rancher's booth. Here, surrounded by photos of cattle and sheep grazing on grass and chickens running around freely, the rancher makes suggestions on what I can make for dinner and gives me recipe advice as well. In the next booth is a vendor selling wild fish that was caught just the day before. Spotting another farmer one booth down, I think about picking up some ears of corn, confident that they will not have come from genetically modified crops.

In July 2008, the New Jersey Supreme Court ruled that factory farming practices cannot be considered humane just because they are commonly and widely used.

The other way to shop (one I try to avoid as much as possible) is going to a supermarket. Above all else, what you really need to know and remember is that almost all of the meat, poultry, and eggs sold in supermarkets in this country come from factory farms, feedlots, or CAFOs (confined animal feeding operations). Most CAFOs pay little attention to human health, food safety, the humane treatment of animals, or the environment. In these over-

Born and Raised in the USA?

As of September 2008, you can now look at a pork chop or a pound of hamburger and see a label that says where it came from. "Country of Origin Labeling," or COOL, on beef, pork, chicken, and lamb will tell you whether the animals were raised in the United States or another country.

crowded industrial settings, animals are fed whatever it takes to grow them as large and as fast as possible. That usually means synthetic growth hormones and feed consisting of grain, corn, and soy (most often genetically modified). According to the Union of Concerned Scientists, "These feeds also contain same species meat, diseased animals, feathers, hair, skin, hooves, blood, plastics, and other animal waste." Since cows are meant to eat grass and not grain, their stomachs become acidic, and they develop ulcers and other digestive problems. Ranchers then dose the cows with antibiotics, which we consumers ingest.

HEALTHIER BEEF

Since the late 1990s, a growing number of ranchers have been letting their cattle graze, which is the diet in harmony with nature. The animals eat nothing but fresh grass and cut hay—and their mothers' milk—their entire lives. They tend to be healthier and more humanely treated.

Grass-fed beef does cost more than conventional beef, so why go out of your way and pay more for it? Cattle that eat grass their entire lives are not given growth hormones or antibiotics, and their meat is higher in omega-3 fatty acids and lower in saturated fat and cholesterol. Plus, "cows, when grazed properly, help reduce CO_2 in the air by increasing soil organic matter," says Allan Nation, publisher of the *Stockman Grass Farmer*, which helps educate cattle farmers about the benefits of grass.

Aside from omega-3s, grass-fed beef contains another beneficial fat called conjugated linoleic acid (CLA). CLA is present in all beef, but a 1999 study that appeared in the *Journal of Dairy Science* found that grass-fed beef had 500 percent more CLA than beef from cows fed a grain-based diet.

You can find grass-fed beef at local farmers' markets, natural food stores, and specialty meat markets. Grass-fed advocates say to look for "100% grass-fed and finished" on the label to be sure.

To save money, consider buying in bulk at a CSA. You can purchase a share, a half or whole animal, or a box of assorted cuts.

If you can't find grass fed beef locally, check out these online sources: www.americangrassfed.org, www.eatwild.com, www.eatwellguide.org, and www.localharvest.org. You also can buy by mail order from sources such as www.hardwickbeef.com, www.LaCenseBeef.com, www.LasaterGrasslandsBeef.com, and www.TallGrassBeef.com.

Grass-Fed Milk

Most cartons of milk in the supermarket show a picture of cows contentedly grazing on grass, but commercial milk comes from cows that ate grain. "Unfortunately, 85 to 95 percent of the cows in the United States are now being raised in confinement, not on pasture," says Jo Robinson, creator of eatwild.com. "The reason for confining our cows in feedlots and feeding them grain rather than grass is that they produce more milk—especially when injected with biweekly hormones. Today's grain-fed cows produce three times as much milk as the old family cow of days gone by."

Commercial milk also can contain residues of the chemicals or drugs used in the feed. These include bovine growth hormone (BGH, also known as BST, rbGH, and rbST), which is genetically engineered and injected into dairy cows so they can produce milk for nearly twice as long after calving. The FDA doesn't require the treated milk to be labeled, so look for organic dairy products or those saying "Does Not Contain Growth Hormones."

Milk from pastured (not pasteurized*) cows appears to be much healthier than conventional milk. In 2008, the United Kingdom *Independent* reported that grass-fed cows offer "60 percent higher levels of conjugated linoleic acid (CLA9), which has been linked to a reduced risk of cancer." Also more abundant in milk from grass-fed cows were omega-3s (39 percent higher) and vitamin E (33 percent higher). Unlike in the United States, the United Kingdom's organic standards make sure that organic milk comes from cows with access to grass when it's abundant in the summer.

To find out where you can buy milk from grass-fed cows, look at eatwild. com's state-by-state directory of farms, which lists more than 800 pasture-based farms.

* The terms pasteurized and ultra-pasteurized *refer to a high-heat process. It is done so manufacturers can sell milk over long distances. Raw-milk advocates claim that the process "kills the milk," destroying its enzymes and many of its vitamins.*

HAPPY CHICKENS AND SPECKLED EGGS

Gone are the days of plucking your own chicken—like my grandmother did—but you can still get good-tasting chickens if you look for those fed on pasture. I've found them at my farmers' market (chicken feet too!), although they cost more than conventional birds. Chickens sold in supermarkets, if not organic, were fed a mixture of conventionally grown (sometimes genetically modified) corn and soy that is often laced with growth hormones and antibiotics. Studies show that eggs from chickens raised on pasture, where they eat grass and insects, are higher in omega-3s and vitamins E and A, and lower in total fat, saturated fat, and cholesterol. Omega-3s account for seven percent of the total fat content of grass-fed beef compared with only one percent of grain-fed beef.

The definition of a "free-range" or "free-roaming" chicken is that the bird has access to the outdoors. This means that the enclosure must have a door, and the door has to be open at least part of the time. It doesn't mean the chickens are actually roaming around on the range freely! For eggs, the term "cage-free" means the egg-laying chickens are not put in small cages but instead are put into big enclosures with no outdoor access.

In 2008, voters in California voted on Proposition 2, which seeks to increase cage sizes for egg-laying hens, pregnant pigs, and veal calves. The new regulations, which go into effect in 2015, require cages to be large enough to allow these animals to be able to stand up, lie down, turn around, and fully extend their limbs without touching the side of an enclosure or other egg-laying hens.

WHAT YOU SHOULD KNOW

- "Organic" means that chickens and cows ate organic feed and were not given antibiotics. Typically, they, too, are raised in confinement. The same is true for chickens and cows fed vegetarian feed (that is, feed that contains no meat by-products).

- "Natural" means no additives or preservatives were introduced after the meat or poultry was processed.

MYTH: "Cage-free" and "free-range" mean "free-roaming" and thus natural, healthy chickens and eggs.

TRUTH: These terms are misleading. The chickens may get a little more room to eat and socialize, but they are still raised on feedlots with unnatural diets.

- Most supermarket eggs are produced with sometimes close to 500,000 birds in one facility, creating inhumane conditions and the need to give chickens drugs to control disease outbreaks.

- Many commercial egg producers add synthetic colorants to their feed to make the yolks a brighter yellow, but no label stating that appears on the carton.

3 WAYS TO MAKE A SHIFT

1. Choose grass-fed or pastured beef and poultry.
2. Buy organic eggs and, if possible, eggs from chickens raised on pasture.
3. Buy organic milk, and, if possible, from cows that ate grass.

Where to Shop

Many farmers' markets and locally owned farms offer fresh eggs from free-roaming chickens and beef that has been raised on a green pasture instead of in a crowded, manure-filled feedlot. Stores such as Whole Foods, Trader Joe's, Safeway, and even Walmart are offering natural beef and chicken as well as wild fish. They also sell eggs with added omega-3s, which are beneficial to your health.

FUTURE FISH

Farmed fish are no better off than farmed chickens and cows. In 1981, I wrote an eerily prophetic article called "Future Fish" for *Savvy*, a now-defunct women's magazine. In it I stated, "Instead of boats on the ocean, the smell of salt air and the soft cry of seagulls, the world of tomorrow's fishermen may be conveyor belts, holding tanks, aeration devices, pumps, filters, and water-analysis kits."

A short 18 years later, the majority of fish sold in most American restaurants and markets are being raised on fish farms, often called "feedlots of the sea," where they are housed in pens with the same overcrowded con-

In the 1970s it took ten weeks to raise a broiler; now it takes 40 days in a dark and crowded shed, because farmers are under constant pressure to cut costs and increase productivity.

—PAUL ROBERTS,
The End of Food

ditions experienced by cattle and chickens. Fish are vaccinated against disease, dosed with antibiotics, and fed pesticides to fend off sea lice. In fact, sea lice from fish farms have become a huge problem—the lice are infecting and killing off young wild salmon that swim by the pens, and their survival, it has been reported, is now at stake.

Don't be fooled by a restaurant or store selling "organic" farmed fish. An organic salmon, for example, doesn't exist in nature. What it means is that the fish was raised in a crowded cage or pen and fed a diet of organic fish food. It will not have a high omega-3 content like its wild counterpart that ate from the sea. While it's true that they are given organic feed, they still are fed coloring to dye their flesh, and are routinely given medicines to prevent sea lice and fungal growth. The uneaten food (organic or not) that falls from the pens covers the sea floor below, which is becoming a big problem for other marine life in the ocean.

"To rid salmon of sea lice, fish farmers spike their feed with a strong pesticide called emamectin benzoate, which when administered to rats and dogs causes tremors, spinal deterioration and muscle atrophy. The farmed salmon in nearly every American supermarket may contain this pesticide, which on land is used to rid diseased trees of pine beetles. It is not a substance I want in my body."

—TARAS GRESCOE, *Bottomfeeder*

Suspicious Shrimp

Shrimp has become a staple in supermarket fish counters, but most of these shrimp are farmed in countries such as Vietnam and Cambodia, and many of the farmers there use chemicals to prevent disease and rapidly increase their growth. According to a 2008 article in London's *Observer*, "The prawns, packed in the ponds, are terribly prone to illness, so they're fed a chemical commonly used as a 'nutritional enhancer' as well as pesticides, feed enhancers and growth stimulants; methyl hydroxybenzoate, an anti-fungal preservative that is banned in France and Australia and has been linked to cancer in some beauty treatments; and norfloxacin, an antibiotic usually used to treat gonorrhea and urinary tract infections in humans."

In his book *Bottomfeeder: How to Eat Ethically in a World of Vanishing*

"Farmed salmon contain higher levels of PCBs, dioxin, flame retardants, pesticides, and other toxins than wild salmon because these contaminants are often present in the fish that are ground up for feed."

—Food & Water Watch

Seafood, Taras Grescoe says he thinks farmed shrimp is the most disgusting of all the industrial farmed products—worse than salmon and battery chicken—and he won't eat them.

Food & Water Watch, a non-profit consumer organization, has studied prawn farming for 10 years. It states in its 2008 report: "The negative effects of eating industrially produced shrimp may include neurological damage from ingesting chemicals such as endosulfans, an allergic response to penicillin residues or infection by an antibiotic-resistant pathogen such as *E coli*."

WHAT YOU SHOULD KNOW

- Farmed-raised salmon are fed synthetic colorants to make the fish's flesh match the orange color of their wild counterparts. Labels on farmed Atlantic salmon must include the words "artificially colored" or "color added."

- According to Canadian and British studies, farmed salmon accumulate more cancer-causing polychlorinated biphenyls (PCBs) and toxic dioxins than wild salmon.

- A staggering 37 percent of all global seafood is now ground up to make fish pellets that feed farmed fish. If things keep going at this rate, our wild fish supply will eventually be nonexistent.

Fish Labels

Look for the blue Marine Stewardship Council (MSC) logo on fish. This tells you that the fish were not overfished or harvested in ways that harm the ocean. The MSC certification is awarded to seafood products that come from sustainable sources—that is, fishing practices that allow a depleted or threatened fish population to recover to healthy levels. These practices also keep healthy fish populations from becoming depleted. For more information, look at the MSC Web site: www.msc.org.

3 WAYS TO MAKE A SHIFT

1. When choosing fish, avoid farmed varieties even if they are labeled as "organic."

2. Choose smaller fish, such as herring, sardines, and mackerel, which are less likely to have toxins than large fish such as tuna or swordfish. They also are very rich in omega-3s.

3. If you must eat farmed fish, nutrition expert Marion Nestle, PhD, author of *Safe Food: Bacteria, Biotechnology, and Bioterrorism,* advises that you broil or grill it until it is well done. Also remove the skin to get rid of much of the toxin-laden grease.

GENETICALLY MODIFIED FOODS, AKA "FRANKENFOODS"

There's something very quiet happening in our food stores. You won't hear it being spoken about by food sellers or find it written on a label. But silently, GMOs, or genetically modified organisms, are infiltrating everyday foods such as flours, cereals, oils, salad dressings, mayonnaise, pies, chips, cookies, fried foods, and even candy coatings.

Genetic engineering, or biotech, generally takes genes from one species and inserts them into the genome of a completely unrelated species using viruses as a carrier. It differs from conventional crop modification and breeding in that it lets scientists (not farmers) achieve results quickly.

Supporters of biotech foods see them as a boon to feeding the hungry and boosting harvests, yet opponents are concerned. Some scientists and food safety advocates have suggested that genetically engineered foods might harm the human immune system, lead to dangerous antibiotic resistance, or result in new and untreatable allergies. In 1996, for example, scientists inserted a Brazil nut gene into a soybean to make the bean more nutritious. The result was a soybean that triggered nut allergies in people, and the Brazil nut–soybean project came to a halt.

In another experiment, in 2000, European scientists announced that by inserting a daffodil gene (and a few other genes) into rice, they created a

By 2015, the United Nations Food and Agriculture Organization expects half of all seafood consumed worldwide to come from farms.

grain with 23 times the beta-carotene of normal rice. The rice, called "Golden Rice," was touted as a solution to vitamin A deficiency, which can cause blindness in developing countries. But critics claimed that the rice couldn't supply enough beta-carotene to combat blindness. The rice experiment is still going on. In April 2008, field trials of Golden Rice began in the Philippines. In October 2008, the Rockefeller Foundation, a philanthropic organization that funded the original work of Golden Rice's engineers, started to help move the project through approval processes in Bangladesh, India, Indonesia, and the Philippines.

Is GM or genetic engineering, safe? No one knows for sure. The problem is that we consumers are unknowingly eating these foods, and there have been only a limited number of safety tests conducted. In 2007, French scientists published results of a reanalysis of the safety data collected by Monsanto, an agricultural company, on a variety of genetically modified corn. Monsanto had stated that the corn was safe, but when the French scientists looked at the data, they found evidence of decreased weight, liver toxicity, and increased levels of blood lipids in rats. Since the jury is still out on what GM could mean for human health and the environment, it's best to eat organic food to be sure you're safe.

There is also disturbing evidence that genetically engineered plants are turning up where they're not wanted. In 2006, the USDA announced that an unapproved variety of genetically engineered long-grain rice had contaminated nonengineered rice fields in five southern US states. This means that if the wind blows seeds from GM crops into a neighboring organic field, for example, the produce in that field could no longer be certified organic.

Even developing countries are wary of GM crops. In his book *Exposed: The Toxic Chemistry of Everyday Products and What's at Stake for American*

In Vitro Meat

By using stem cells, researcher Jason Matheny, MPH, MBA, a biologist at Johns Hopkins University, and founder of New Harvest, is hoping to produce meat without using animals. He and a consortium of international scientists are investigating ways to grow meat in a lab. They believe that it will eliminate the environmental impact of raising livestock and that the meat would be healthier and could be nutritionally enhanced with substances such as omega-3s.

Power, author Mark Schapiro writes that when a food crisis swept southern Africa, "Zambia and Zimbabwe refused the US offer of corn and soybean donations out of fear they would introduce genetically engineered material into their own agriculture (and thus, also, eliminate them forever from contention as future exporters to Europe)."

Remember, food manufacturers are taking food and inserting a virus in its cells to alter the DNA of a plant. Do you really want to be eating these foods?

WHAT YOU SHOULD KNOW

- GM foods are not labeled, yet more than 60 percent of processed foods on your grocery store shelves contain genetically engineered ingredients! These include many breakfast cereals; pancake, muffin, and cake mixes; salad dressings and margarines; veggie burgers; cookies, chocolate, and tortilla chips; and infant formulas.

- They come from mainly three crops—corn, soy, and canola—and more than 70 GM crops are approved for the marketplace, including some potatoes, cotton, tomatoes, squash, radicchio, and papayas, and many more await commercial approval. They are engineered to do two things: hold up to sprayings of herbicides and resist pests.

- There is insufficient knowledge of the health risks and long-term environmental impacts associated with GM foods.

- Major retail outlets and supermarket chains across Europe will not sell GM foods. Parts of Italy, Poland, and Austria are now GMO-free.

- Concerns about the safety of GM foods has prompted several US towns and counties (mostly in California) to become GMO-free. GMOs also can't be grown in Montville or Maine or on city land in Boulder, Colorado.

3 WAYS TO MAKE A SHIFT

1. Just say no to GMOs!
2. Start looking for labels that say "No GMOs," or choose organic, which by law cannot be genetically modified. Also check the PLU (price look-up) number on the stickers of fruits and vegetables. Conventionally grown produce has four numbers; organically grown has five numbers prefaced by

the number 9; GMO produce has five numbers prefaced by the number 8. (Example: a conventionally grown Fuji apple is 4131; organic is 94131; GMO is 84131.)

3. Avoid nonorganic corn and soy products, since these will most likely contain GMOs.

Foods Most Likely to Contain GMOs

- Corn: The #1 American agricultural commodity. 25% is genetically engineered.

- Soy: The #2 US agricultural commodity. Sixty percent of processed foods contain soy ingredients, and 82% of edible fats and oils are soy-based. 54% is genetically engineered.

- Canola oil: Of the 15 million acres of canola grown in the United States and Canada annually, 35% are genetically engineered.

- Cottonseed oil: Every year, half a million tons of cottonseed oil go into salad dressings, baked goods, and snack foods.

- Papaya: More than one third of Hawaiian papayas have been genetically engineered to withstand the papaya ringspot virus. Organic papaya grow-

And Candy, Too?

In 2008, US farmers planted GM sugar beet crops for the first time. The beets are genetically altered to survive regular applications of Monsanto's weed killer, Roundup, and its active ingredient, glyphosate, considered a toxic herbicide. Citizens for Health, a nonprofit consumer advocacy group, says, "Since half of the granulated sugar in the US comes from sugar beets, the infiltration of GE (GM) sugar beets represents a significant alteration of our food supply." Since US law does not require labeling of GM ingredients, when we buy products such as candy or Kellogg's breakfast cereal we will unknowingly be exposed to engineered sugar, with unknown health consequences. In addition, the European Union has not approved GE sugar beets for human consumption. To find out more or to take action against GE foods, go to the Organic Consumer's Web site: www. organicconsumers.org.

ers in Hawaii worry that the pollen from GE papaya trees will contaminate their crops.

- Salmon: A company called Aqua Bounty has engineered a salmon with genes from two different fish species so that it grows much more quickly than non-GE salmon. The company is now seeking FDA approval to market this fish for human consumption.

Source: Healthy Child Healthy World Organization

UNSUNG HERO

Allan Nation is a pioneer at the forefront of grass farming in America. Allan teaches farmers and ranchers to become extremely successful at increasing the gross output of their land by raising cattle on grass rather than in feedlots. He suggests that farmers should focus on local markets, rely on reputation and word of mouth, and above all rely as much as possible on free solar energy rather than fossil fuels to feed their livestock.

Allan, the son of a commercial cattle rancher, grew up in Greenville, Mississippi. He became the agricultural reporter for his local newspaper at age 16. He has traveled to over 30 countries around the world studying and photographing grassland farming systems. Since 1977, he has been the editor of *The Stockman Grass Farmer* magazine, the only monthly publication in North America devoted solely to management-intensive grassland farming in all its aspects. In 1993 he received the Agricultural Conservation Award from the American Farmland Trust for spearheading the drive behind the grass farming revolution in the United States.

Allan is the author of eight books, including *Knowledge Rich Ranching*, *Quality Pasture*, and *Grassfed to Finish*. For more information, go to his Web site: www.stockmangrassfarmer.net.

Chapter 4

UNFILTERED TAP WATER

Don't Take Clean Water for Granted, Plus the Possible Peril of Plastic

"Not all chemicals are bad. Without chemicals such as hydrogen and oxygen, for example, there would be no way to make water, a vital ingredient in beer."

—Dave Barry

As a child growing up in the 1960s in Queens, New York, I used to drink clean, clear water from my kitchen faucet. But times have changed. If you think the water coming out of your tap is clean and health-giving, you'd be mistaken. In 2003, the NRDC (Natural Resources Defense Council) reviewed the tap water quality in all American cities; their report revealed the presence of several contaminants—including chlorination by-products, lead, coliform bacteria, and industrial chemicals—in the water supplies of many cities, with Atlanta, Albuquerque, San Francisco, and Fresno having fair-to-substandard drinking water.

More recently, in 2008, an investigation by the Associated Press showed that America's tap water, coast to coast, is contaminated with a vast array of prescription and over-the-counter drugs, including antibiotics, pain medications, antidepressants, and sex hormones. This is happening because when people take pills, their bodies absorb some of the medication, but the rest is flushed down the toilet, and water treatment plants don't remove pharmaceutical residues.

They remain in the water that eventually lands back in our drinking water supplies.

Scientists are concerned that even in small concentrations these drugs could harm us over time because water is consumed in such large amounts every day. Our bodies may be able to deal with a big one-time dose of a chemical, but if a small amount is consumed continuously over years . . . no one really knows what can happen to our health. Also, there's no national strategy to deal with this issue. There are "no effective mandates to test, treat, limit or even advise the public," reports the Associated Press.

Since we can't live without water (it's a vital component of our bodies, making up about 70 percent of our muscles and brain tissue), it's critical to drink only clean, pure water. In addition, health authorities now agree that fluoride, added to most tap water, should not be given to infants. Go to www. fluoridealert.org.

WHAT YOU SHOULD KNOW

- A chemical pollutant from rocket fuel called perchlorate has been detected in many US water sources and could harm nursing babies. According to a team at the Albert Einstein College of Medicine, New York, and the Johns Hopkins School of Medicine, Baltimore, perchlorate becomes concentrated in breast milk.

- According to the US Geological Survey and Associated Press, municipal drinking water typically contains 100 or so pharmaceutical medicines (including narcotics and oral contraceptives) in "significant concentrations."

- The United Nations Educational, Scientific and Cultural Organization (UNESCO) reports that up to 500 million tons of heavy metals, solvents, and toxic sludge slip into the global water supply every year.

- According to the Earth Day Network, 14 million people in the United States now regularly drink water contaminated with chemicals known to cause cancer.

- The Worldwatch Institute declared that toxic chemicals from hazardous liquid waste (34 billion liters of solvents, heavy metals, and radioactive materials per year) are contaminating much of the groundwater in the United States.

What's on Tap

To check your local water quality: go to the Natural Resources Defense Council's Web site at www.nrdc.org, find the "Issues" page, then click on "Water." From there you should be able to access your community's Annual Quality Report. You also can ask your water utility company for a copy of its annual water quality report, or call the Environmental Protection Agency's (EPA's) Safe Drinking Water Hotline at 800-426-4791. Your own water could be further contaminated because of old pipes leading to your faucets, making it even more important to use a good-quality water filter.

To get your water tested: use a company such as National Testing Laboratories Ltd., which is a network of certified laboratories that analyzes drinking water according to the EPA's methods. Call 800-458-3330 to check for lead or to get a comprehensive screening. To find other labs, check the NRDC Web site: www.nrdc.org.

3 WAYS TO MAKE A SHIFT

1. Learn what's in your tap. Call your local water utility and request a copy of your community's annual water quality report.

2. Buy a water filter (see below for recommendations) and fill up your own reusable water bottles, preferably stainless steel or glass, at home.

3. Ditch your polycarbonate water bottles (marked #7 on the bottom) in favor of a stainless steel bottle. If there's a hint of the smell or taste of plastic in your water, don't drink it. Instead, store water in glass or brass if possible and out of direct sunlight.

FILTERED AND PURIFIED WATER

Filtering or purifying your own tap water is the most economical and probably the healthiest solution in the long run. Knowing which type of filter or apparatus to use is more challenging. It's not easy to make sense of all the different water filters on the market or to be confident about the quality claims manufacturers make. Here's an overview of the devices and techniques that are available.

Another Reason to Test Your Water

Reduced-flush toilets, low-flow shower heads, and other well-intentioned water conservation efforts are allowing water to remain in household pipes longer, according to Marc Edwards, PhD, a professor at Virginia Tech University and an authority on the quality of drinking water. In 2008, Dr. Edwards reported in the *American Chemical Society Journal on Environmental Science and Technology*, "As water stagnates in pipes, it can develop bacteria and [have] other unwanted effects on household plumbing."

Simple filtration: This is a relatively inexpensive method in which tap water passes through a fine strainer and/or activated carbon or charcoal (the popular Brita and Pur water systems are good examples). While it can remove unpleasant odors and tastes, it doesn't completely remove many common contaminants, such as bacteria, viruses, parasites, lead, arsenic, copper, nitrates, and chloramines (a chlorine-ammonia combination that's being added to more and more municipal water supplies around the country). Chloramines are corrosive and will slowly dissolve metals such as lead and copper from your pipes, raising their levels in your drinking water.

A new Brita-type water filter on the market, called ZeroWater (www.zerowater.com), claims to remove lead, iron, zinc and mercury as well as antibiotics, hormones, and perchlorate. The units are made of styrene and are free of bisphenol A.

Purification: A purifier is defined as a device that removes 90 to 95 percent of all contaminants in water. There are three main purifier technologies: reverse osmosis, steam distillation, and ultraviolet disinfection. These systems have to be installed, generally under your kitchen sink or at the water source to the whole house, which is more expensive. Companies around the country sell water purification systems (see the Recommended Resources section).

- **Reverse osmosis:** High pressure forces water through a semi-permeable membrane to trap toxins. These systems vary greatly in their ability to rid water of contaminants. Their performance level depends on numerous factors, including pH, water temperature and pressure, dissolved solids, and the initial water contaminant level. It gets rid of most contaminants, including parasites such as *Giardia*; heavy metals such as lead and mercury; and pollutants such as arsenic. It's used often in combination with a carbon filter.

- **Steam distillation:** This type of system boils water and uses evaporation and condensation to separate water from its contaminants. Certain devices on the market claim that distillation, combined with carbon filtration, provides the greatest reduction in contaminants, including biological elements as well as heavy metals and arsenic. However, it's been shown that the more distilled water a person drinks, the more acidic the body can become. An acid environment in the body can be a breeding ground for diseases such as cancer.

- **Ultraviolet disinfection:** Ultraviolet light removes harmful bacteria, viruses, and microorganisms, as well as chlorine, polychlorinated biphenyls, lead, ethylene dibromide, trichloroethylene, trihalomethanes, tetradecylcyclobutanone, and 50 more chemical contaminants and pesticides that are on the EPA's Primary Health Related Contaminants list for drinkable water. Some think that the water dispensed from an ultraviolet filtration system is about the healthiest water you can possibly drink.

GET OFF PLASTIC BOTTLES

If you've switched to bottled water in hopes of avoiding the perils of drinking tap water, consider this: Eight out of 10 plastic water bottles used in the United States become garbage or end up in a landfill, contributing to global warming. They're also found in our oceans as small bits of plastic that fish and birds mistakenly eat because they look like krill. Greenpeace says a single 1-liter drink bottle could break down into enough small fragments to put one on every mile of beach in the entire world.

Plastic debris is a huge problem. A sea of plastic has formed in an area of the Pacific Ocean known as the North Pacific Gyre. It has been described as a plastic soup twice the size of Texas. It's estimated that over a million sea-birds and 100,000 marine mammals and sea turtles are killed each year by ingestion of plastics.

More than half of all Americans drink bottled water; about a third of us consume it regularly, paying from 240 to over 10,000 times more per gallon than we do for tap water. Sales of bottled water have tripled in the past 10 years to about $4 billion per year, and the environmental impact is enormous. Every year, 1.5 million tons of plastic are used in bottled water manufacturing.

It is up to us to avoid plastic in the things we buy and to recycle our plastic bottles when we do use them.

Part of the reason people buy water in plastic bottles is their concerns about the hazards of most tap water. But is bottled water any safer? In a major study conducted by the NRDC comparing 1,000 bottles of different brands of water, several of the brands were shown to contain dangerous chemicals. Here are a few of their disturbing findings:

- About one-third of the bottled water tested positive for significant chemical or bacterial contamination, exceeding levels allowed under a state or industry standard or guideline.

- The longer a bottle of water sits on a shelf, whether in a grocery store or your refrigerator, the more likely you are to consume a larger dose of a chemical called antimony, a potential carcinogen that leaches from the plastic.

Buying a Water Filter

The best protection for your health is a whole-house water filter, although it is the most expensive option. This system is attached to the incoming cold water line of your home, so all the taps in the house dispense clean water. It's always a good idea to use a local dealer who is familiar with the water quality in your area when choosing a unit—whether it's an under-the-sink or whole-house system.

According to the NRDC, when choosing a water filter do these three things:

1. Make sure you get a filter that removes the contaminants of concern in your tap water. (See your city's annual water quality report for information, or NRDC's report at www.nrdc.org)

2. Be sure the filter is independently certified by NSF International (or a similar independent organization) to remove the contaminants of concern in your tap water (1800-NSF-MARK).

3. Maintain the filter at least as often as the manufacturer recommends, or hire a maintenance company to maintain it for you.

Check the Recommended Resources for online sources of water filters.

- About one-fifth of the bottled water contained industrial or manufacturing chemicals such as toluene, xylene, phthalate, adipate, and styrene. If these contaminants are consumed over a long period of time, they might cause cancer or other health problems.

It is estimated that about 25 to 30 percent of the bottled water sold in the United States comes from a city or town's tap water—sometimes further treated, sometimes not. To find out if your bottled water comes from city tap water, check the label or the cap. If it says "from a municipal source" or "from a community water system," it's derived from tap water.

The Environmental Working Group conducted a study of bottled water in 2008 and found 38 pollutants in 24 samples from 10 major brands purchased by the group in California, Washington, DC, and eight other states. Some of the substances they uncovered were caffeine, Tylenol, arsenic, radioactive isotopes, nitrates, ammonia from fertilizer residue, as well as industrial chemicals used as solvents, degreasing agents, and propellants.

In addition, bottled water may contain chemicals (such as antimony, mentioned above) that can leach out of plastic bottles, made of PET, or polyethylene terephthalate. Microwaving a bottle or leaving it in the sun or a hot car can accelerate the process.

While the bottled water industry maintains that there are no chemical contaminants in bottled water, the NRDC determined that "one cannot assume on faith, simply because one is buying water in a bottle, that the water is of any higher chemical quality than tap water."

BPA in Plastic

BPA (bisphenol-A) is a chemical that acts a lot like estrogen when it's introduced into the body. It can get there by leaching out of hard plastic bottles as they age, are heated (in microwave ovens or dishwashers), or are exposed to acidic solutions. The Centers for Disease Control and Prevention discovered BPA in 93 percent of children and adults tested in the United States between 2003 and 2004.

Frederick vom Saal, PhD, a biology professor at the University of Missouri–Columbia and one of the leading BPA researchers in the country, reports that in studies of laboratory animals, BPA changes play behavior, weakens gender differences, decreases sperm count, stimulates prostate cancer, and causes symptoms of attention-deficit hyperactivity disorder. Dr. vom Saal believes that BPA should be banned from all products.

The United Nations has declared
2005 to 2015 "Water for Life," the
International Decade for Action on
water-related issues.

There is a strong push to eliminate BPA around the world. In 2006 Europe banned all BPA-containing products made for children under age 3, and in December of that year San Francisco did the same. In March 2007 a billion-dollar class action suit was started in Los Angeles superior court against Gerber Playtex, Evenflo, Avent, and Dr. Brown's for harm done to babies caused by drinking out of baby bottles and sippy cups containing BPA.

In October 2008, America's third largest grocery chain, Safeway, announced that it will stop selling plastic baby bottles made with BPA. Whole Foods, Walmart, and Toys R Us have done the same, with many more retailers and manufacturers sure to follow. Until they do, it's probably best to follow Dr. vom Saal's advice: "If it's hard and clear and [it] doesn't say 'No BPA,' don't use it."

3 WAYS TO MAKE A SHIFT

1. Buy tomato sauce in glass jars. Canned tomato sauce is likely to have higher levels of BPA because the high acidity of the tomatoes causes more of the chemical to leach from the lining of the can.

2. Purchase beverages in plastic or glass bottles. Canned soda and juice often contain some BPA.

3. If you opt to use plastic kitchenware, get rid of the older, scratched-up ones and avoid putting them in the dishwasher, since these things can cause more chemicals to leach into your food.

WATER ON THE GO

Now, if you've decided to filter your own water and fill up your own reusable bottles, which bottles are best? Stainless steel or aluminum should be your first choice, but if you must use plastic, make certain that the bottle won't leach. You can do this by checking the recycling symbol on the bottom of the bottle. If you see a #2 HDPE (high-density polyethylene), a #4 LDPE (low-density polyethylene), or a #5 PP (polypropylene), the bottle is fine. The type of plastic bottle in which water and soft drinks are usually sold is a #1. While it is considered safe, it is recommended for one-time use only. In other words, do not refill it—it makes a good breeding ground for bacteria.

Plastics to Avoid

- #3 Polyvinyl chloride (PVC) contains the phthalate DEHP [di(2-ethylhexyl) phthalate], an endocrine disruptor and probable human carcinogen.

- #6 Polystyrene (PS) may leach styrene, a possible endocrine disruptor and human carcinogen.

BPA in Cans, Too!

Besides plastic bottles, BPA is found in the epoxy resins used as a coating in metal food and beverage cans to prevent the metal from coming into contact with the food contents and to help those contents flow out easily. About 85 percent of the food cans sold in the United States have plastic linings.

When the Environmental Working Group tested canned food for BPA contamination, it found that a single serving from one in 10 cans of all food, and one in three cans of infant formula, contained enough BPA to expose people to levels more than 200 times the government's traditional safe level of exposure for industrial chemicals. Of all foods tested, chicken soup, infant formula, and ravioli had the highest BPA levels. In 2005, researchers from Yale School of Medicine reported that low doses of BPA may lead to learning disabilities and age-related neurodegenerative diseases in humans. In a 2008 follow-up study, Yale School of Medicine linked BPA to problems with brain function and mood disorders in monkeys, reaffirming that low-dose exposure to the chemical can have negative effects on the brain and hormonal system.

Bottom line? Choose foods in glass jars whenever possible. If you do eat foods from cans, seek out companies that claim not to use BPA. These include Trader Joe's, Eden Foods, Westbrook Farms, and Bionaturae. Several major retailers, including Walmart and Toys R Us, have pledged to drop BPA products in 2009, while some makers of baby bottles and sports bottles have switched to BPA-free plastic. If you're formula feeding your infant, consider using powdered formulas packaged in nonsteel cans.

Types of Water to Drink

Here's an explanation of several different types of water. Personally, I prefer to drink the first three on the list since they are the most natural and least treated.

- Spring water: This originates from an underground spring or well. Most springs are protected to keep them pure, yet natural impurities such as arsenic, fluoride, radon, and uranium may be present. Spring water may be flat (still) or carbonated.

- Artesian water: This originates from an aquifer, a deep underground flow of water. It can contain some contaminants.

- Mineral: This water contains dissolved minerals (mostly calcium and magnesium), which are either naturally occurring or added at a bottling plant. Fluoride may be present.

- Sparkling water: This water is naturally carbonated, though most brands add carbonation due to the loss of the natural "fizz" during processing. Many have high levels of fluoride.

- Distilled: this is water that has been vaporized; all minerals and chemicals have been removed.

- Fluoridated: Over half of American water treatment plants add fluoride to prevent cavities. Fluoride is controversial and is suspected of being a health hazard, and many European countries have banned its use.

- Chlorinated: Chlorine is added to 70 percent of municipal water supplies. It destroys bacteria, including those that result in typhoid fever, cholera, and dysentery. Chlorine is also suspected of being hazardous to our health.

- Boiled: boiling kills bacteria in water, but does not remove chemicals such as chlorine or fluoride.

- Alkaline: This type of water has a pH of 7.4 or higher. It is said to help balance the body's pH, which can be acidic from eating things such as sugar and processed foods. There are systems on the market that can alkalinize your drinking water, but be aware that you can become over-alkaline, so it's important to test your pH levels. You can find pH test strips at Amazon.cm

#7 Polycarbonate—those fabulous colorful hard plastic bottles—may leach BPA as bottles age, are heated, or are exposed to acidic solutions. #7 is used in most baby bottles, sippy cups, 5-gallon water jugs, and many reusable sports bottles.

Plastics that are okay to use (check the numbers on bottoms of bottles): #2 HDPE, #4 LDPE, #5 PP, and #1 once. Remember this handy saying from the Institute for Agriculture and Trade Policy: "With your food, use 4, 5, 1, and 2. All the rest aren't good for you."

Safe Water Bottles

Stainless steel: Unlike plastic, these bottles can handle a variety of liquids, including acidic fruit juices, and won't leach chemicals into your beverage. Look for those made with 304, sanitary-grade, or surgical-grade stainless steel to ensure high-quality. Good options include:

- Klean Kanteen bottles, which are constructed from high-quality, food-grade stainless steel. They are easy to clean, durable, and fruit- and acidic-beverage safe.

- Earthlust's unlined, double-walled bottles, which are made from food-grade stainless steel and decorated with nontoxic paints. They are fruit- and acidic-beverage safe.

Aluminum: These are very lightweight, and some are coated on the interior with a permanent epoxy resin that contains no plastic or leaching materials. Good options include:

- Sigg bottles, which are extrusion-pressed from a single, seamless piece of aluminum and are considered the "world's toughest water bottle." They are lined with a nontoxic epoxy, have been thoroughly tested to ensure 0.0% leaching, and exceed all FDA requirements. They are fruit- and acidic-beverage safe and Swiss made (except cold/hot style) since 1908.

- Laken bottles, which have an aluminum exterior process similar to the Sigg bottles and feature a powder coating on the exterior that provides extra protection from wear-and-tear. The FDA-approved epoxy interior prevents leaching and protects beverages. They are fruit- and acidic-beverage safe and Spanish made since 1912.

Eastman Tritan copolyester: It may look like a traditional plastic water bottle, but the brand-new polymer is completely BPA-free and offers superior chemical, heat, and detergent resistance. A good option is the CamelBak water bottle, which is completely BPA-free and has excellent impact resistance. It's suitable for both warm and cold beverages and is dishwasher safe, as well as fruit- and acidic-beverage safe.

Glass: If you'd like to drink water from a great-looking, earth-friendly bottle supercharged with a little love, try the Love Bottle. It's a reusable glass water bottle made from 100% recycled glass. It has a ceramic swing top lid that creates a water-tight seal. Every printed bottle has the word "love" on it (charging your water with the energy of love*), or you can customize your bottle by writing or drawing anything you like on it. The Love Bottle can be found at Whole Foods and Bed Bath & Beyond, and online at: www.lovebottle.net.

For babies, choose tempered glass or opaque plastic made of polypropylene (#5), which does not contain BPA.

THE BOTTOM LINE

When you're dehydrated, any drinkable water is better than no water at all. But when you want optimum health, choose pure, clean water—either filtered or purified in your home—or buy natural spring, artesian, or mineral water. Also, make sure you choose a bottle that's made of safe, nontoxic materials to keep both you and your water healthy.

UNSUNG HERO

In 2002, philanthropist, industrialist, and environmentalist **Jin Zidell** of northern California created the Blue Planet Run Foundation to address the world's water crisis. About one in five people on our planet does not have daily, immediate access to safe drinking water. Instead of just going to the kitchen tap or a water cooler anytime you're thirsty, imagine having to hoist a heavy vessel onto your head and walk up to 2 hours to a well, filling the vessel, and then carrying it for up to 2 more hours back home. This is the

---

* Words and pictures carry energy that affects water, says the Japanese researcher Dr. Masaru Emoto, chief of the Hado institute in Tokyo and author of *The Hidden Messages in Water*. To learn more about his work and to view photographs of water crystals, visit www.hado.net.

What the Recycling Numbers Mean

#1—PET or PETE (polyethylene terephthalate). Found in: Soft drink, water, and beer bottles; mouthwash bottles; peanut butter containers; salad dressing and vegetable oil containers. It poses low risk of leaching; intended for one-time use.

#2—HDPE (high-density polyethylene). Found in: Milk jugs; juice bottles; bleach, detergent, and household cleaner bottles; shampoo bottles; some trash and shopping bags; butter and yogurt tubs; cereal box liners. It carries low risk of leaching and is recyclable into many goods.

#3—V (Vinyl) or PVC. Found in: Window cleaner and detergent bottles, shampoo bottles, cooking oil bottles, clear food packaging. PVC contains chlorine, so its manufacture can release highly dangerous dioxins. Don't use in the microwave!

#4—LDPE (low-density polyethylene). Found in: Squeezable bottles, bread bags, frozen food bags, shopping bags, tote bags. It carries low risk of leaching.

#5—PP (polypropylene). Found in: Some yogurt containers, syrup bottles, ketchup bottles, bottle caps, straws. It has a high melting point, and so is often used for containers that accept hot liquid. Contains no BPA; considered nonleaching.

#6—PS (polystyrene). Found in: Disposable plates and cups, meat trays, egg cartons, carry-out containers, aspirin bottles. It can be made into rigid or foam products, such as Styrofoam. Evidence suggests it can leach toxins into foods.

#7—Miscellaneous. Found in: Three- and five-gallon water bottles, certain food containers. Polycarbonate is #7, and is found in the hard plastic bottles that studies prove leach hormone disruptors, especially when heated.

dilemma facing hundreds of millions of women and children in Africa, Afghanistan, India, and other parts of Asia, and Central and South America each day.

Jin's mission: to provide safe drinking water to 200 million people for the rest of their lives by 2027. Since 2004, the foundation has funded 18 nongovernmental organizations worldwide, which in turn have implemented 142 sustainable water projects in 14 countries, affecting 137,000 people. The foundation's fundraising event is the Blue Planet Run, the first-ever around-the-world relay run.

For the latest updates and sources for clean water and organic, pasture-raised, and wild food sources, visit www.supernaturalhome.com.

For more information, go to: www.BluePlanetRun.org.

What Goes *on* You

How to Choose Safe Cosmetics and Body Care Products

"Beauty, to me, is about being comfortable in your own skin. That, or a kick-ass red lipstick."

—GWYNETH PALTROW

THE FIRST TIME I truly became aware of the staggering amount of body care products and cosmetics we use on a daily basis was in the locker room at my gym a few years ago. I was heading to the shower after my dance class, and coincidentally, a woman using the locker next to mine was doing the same. She was carrying a basket filled to the brim with shampoo, conditioner, liquid soap, and shaving cream. When I returned to my locker to get dressed, I couldn't help but notice that this same woman was now sitting on a bench where she was pulling bottles and tubes out of another basket in front of her.

First she sprayed antiperspirant under her arms. Then she slathered herself with a heavily scented body lotion, followed by a moisturizer and sunscreen for her face, arms, and chest. Hair care products were next: mousse, some type of shine-enhancer, holding spray.

She then moved on to an array of makeup—foundation, concealer, and blush, followed by eyeliner, two or three eye shadows, and mascara. Finally, lipstick, then gloss. But wait, she wasn't done! She propped one leg up on a stool and began to paint her toenails, first with a clear base, followed by two coats of bright red. Then she opened a third bottle and painted on a quick dry coat. For her finale, she spritzed herself with a hefty dose of perfume.

I became transfixed as I watched this woman's routine, trying not to stare. "Wow!" I thought to myself. "Do most people use this much stuff?" I apply maybe one-third that amount on myself each day, but come to think of it, I never actually took time to read labels or pay attention to what was in the products I put on my skin. I never considered whether these products were safe to use or what effect they might have on my body.

The average consumer uses 15 to 25 cosmetic and personal care products a day. No one really knows what happens in our bodies when we repeatedly expose ourselves to minute amounts of synthetic chemicals from a variety of sources. By the time you walk out of your bathroom in the morning, you may have created a chemical cocktail inside you that is hazardous to your health.

One reason is that your skin is more permeable than you think. It absorbs substances such as medicine from a transdermal patch. This means it also can absorb things that are bad for you, such as preservatives, dyes, and other synthetic chemicals that are in our cosmetics and body care products. These chemicals are literally getting under your skin, where they could be doing damage—even though you can't necessarily "see" it happening. They can lodge in your cells and tissues, and eventually, they might compromise your immune system. A weakened immune system can't do its job of defending you against disease. Many

> **MYTH:** The skin is our barrier organ. It won't let anything bad get past it!
>
> **TRUTH:** While it's true the skin acts like a container to hold in our insides, by no means is it made of concrete. Much to the contrary, it's more like a tightly woven fabric, seemingly impervious but porous at the microscopic level. And chemicals work on a microscopic level.

people falsely believe that they can handle the onslaught of chemicals they're exposed to because the liver will flush them out of the body. This is not necessarily true. Scientists are not certain what the health implications are.

Also, as you read chapters 5 and 6, keep in mind that 98 percent of more than 23,000 skin care and cosmetic products on the market contain one or more ingredients never evaluated for safety by the FDA, CIR (Cosmetic Ingredient Review), or any other publicly accountable institution.

In January 2007, California became the first state to require manufacturers of cosmetic products to disclose the presence of any ingredient known to cause cancer or birth defects. But the rest of the country has no such laws.

That's why environmental groups such as Greenpeace, Friends of the Earth, Teens for Safe Cosmetics, and the Women's Environmental Network (WEN) are complaining that skin creams, shampoos, perfumes, and other cosmetics and toiletries contain chemicals that the human body cannot flush out. They claim the chemicals bioaccumulate, a process by which contaminants gradually collect and increase in concentration in our tissues. There is evidence that this could be harmful. Health advocacy groups assert that when it comes to chemicals that affect human health and the environment, "better safe than sorry" should be the guiding principle.

"Women face daily and widespread exposure to hundreds of chemicals linked to breast cancer, and reducing—or even understanding—this environmental contamination might do as much as screening or treatment to reduce a woman's risk of getting the cancer."

—Report in the May 2007 issue of the journal *Cancer* by Susan G. Komen for the Cure and the Silent Spring Institute

Chapter 5

WHAT'S IN YOUR COSMETICS

And How to Choose Safe Ones

"Cosmetics is a boon to every woman, but a girl's best beauty aid is still a near-sighted man."

—YOKO ONO

"**NATURAL COSMETICS?** They don't work!" "They're just for granola-type women." "There are no natural stores near where I live, so where would I buy them?"

Comments like these are pretty commonplace; they show that there's a lot of resistance to buying natural cosmetics. I've encountered two types of people who have had trouble making the switch. My friend Kathy is a good example of one type. When I first met her, she was the greenest person I knew. She took her own shopping bags to the market before it was fashionable; she drove a hybrid car, ate organic food, and bought her fruits and vegetables from a CSA (community-supported agriculture) farm; she used nontoxic, environmentally friendly household cleaners. But when I asked her if she used natural makeup, she replied, "I don't, and I'm never switching my foundation! It works for me… it covers the sun damage on my face." She totally shut herself off from hearing about any alternative products.

Then there are people like my friend Margaret, who thinks women shouldn't wear any makeup at all because it is unhealthy. By not wearing any herself, she says she's making a statement to others and setting an example. But to me, she looks tired and frumpy—like someone who doesn't care about her appearance.

There is a third way to go, and that is to choose natural cosmetics.

Makeup has been around for centuries, though not the kind we put on ourselves today. Modern makeup tends to be chemically based and to a large extent has never been tested for safety. Out of all those expensive perfumes at the department store beauty counter, for example, almost none uses natural essences. They're made from chemicals rather than flowers. If you've ever walked into an empty room or an elevator and you could still smell the cologne of someone who'd left, you can bet that it was a synthetic fragrance. Unlike natural flower essences, synthetic chemicals have a strong, long-lasting smell.

Many untested chemicals that we put on our skin go *in* our skin as well. Some of the chemicals found in makeup and skin creams are the very same ones used in industrial manufacturing to soften plastics, clean equipment, and stabilize pesticides. One group, known as endocrine disrupters, can work in subtle ways to disrupt the body's ability to produce adequate quantities of hormones or to interfere with the body's hormonal pathways.

The endocrine system regulates every function of the body. It consists of the thyroid, pituitary, and adrenal glands; the pancreas; and the ovaries and the testes, all of which are linked to the hypothalamus in the brain. The hypothalamus sends instructions to the glands to produce hormones. And it is hormones that have a commanding role in how we feel—tired, sad, moody, sexual, hungry, thirsty, and so on. One hormone, estrogen, is secreted by the ovaries and plays a major part in menstruation, fertility, and pregnancy.

Hormones also drive sexual maturation. As girls blossom into young women, could their use of makeup be a factor in their health later in life? A 2005 cosmetic industry report revealed that girls are starting to use cosmetics earlier and more often. Among the report's key findings: 90 percent of 14-year-old girls wear makeup; 63 percent of 7- to 10-year-olds wear lip gloss; and more than two in five girls in the latter age group wear eye shadow or eyeliner. Chances are the glittery lip gloss and eye shadow that moms nonchalantly throw into their daughters' birthday party favor bags contain unhealthy chemicals such as parabens, phthalates, artificial fragrances, and dyes. Because girls are starting to wear makeup so early in life, they may be exposing themselves to these substances for longer periods, which can have a negative impact on their hormones.

At a recent Teens for Safe Cosmetics Summit in Marin County, California, young girls (mostly in high school, but some younger) learned firsthand

> **MYTH:** Any beauty product you buy over the counter or in a department store is safe. The government wouldn't let a company sell a product that potentially could be harmful.
>
> **TRUTH:** There is no regulatory safety board for cosmetics. In fact, claims made on products don't have to meet any standard. So while you may think you're getting a "clinically proven" wrinkle-fighting cream that will take 10 years off your face, you could be applying ingredients to your skin that do more harm than good.

about what was in their makeup. They were asked to bring one of their favorite beauty products to the weekend-long event and trade it in for a healthier version. As one high school junior put it, "I was really surprised to learn about all the bad stuff in the things I use. I thought if a company sells it, it should be safe. When you find out there's so much stuff they're not telling you about, it's scary." It's terrific for girls to get this message at a young age; it might be a good idea for us adults to take heed as well.

As amazing as it may sound, the FDA doesn't review cosmetic ingredients for their safety before they hit the market. An industry-funded panel, known as the Cosmetic Ingredient Review (CIR), not a government health agency, reviews the safety of cosmetic ingredients in the United States. With that in mind, the Environmental Working Group, a nonprofit environmental research organization, assessed more than 23,000 products and found that nearly 1 in every 30 products sold in the United States fails to meet one or more cosmetic safety standards. According to the FDA's Web site (www.fda.gov), "The FDA strongly urges cosmetic manufacturers to conduct whatever toxicological or other tests are appropriate to substantiate the safety of their cosmetics." Translation: It is up to the manufacturers themselves to determine what's safe!

The Environmental Working Group also discovered that nearly 400 products sold in the United States contain chemicals that are unsafe and are prohibited for use in cosmetics in other countries. The 27-country European Union (EU), which includes Germany, France, Italy, and the United Kingdom, recently passed a law banning the use of suspected CMRs—carcinogens, mutagens, or reproductive toxins—in any cosmetics. The major US cosmetics companies that sell abroad—such as L'Oreal, Revlon, and Unilever—have had to reformulate their products to conform to EU safety guidelines. But most haven't changed their formulas for the US market.

More than 1,000 companies have signed the Compact for Safe Cosmetics, a pledge to remove carcinogens and other harmful ingredients from beauty products. The pledge was created by the Campaign for Safe Cosmetics, a coalition of public health, educational, environmental, and consumer groups working in communities, with lawmakers, and directly with cosmetic manufacturers to encourage reformulations and safer ingredients.

All the signers are natural products companies; not one major conventional cosmetic company is on the list. As of this writing, Estee Lauder, L'Oreal, Revlon, Proctor & Gamble, and Unilever have refused to sign. Even Avon, the self-proclaimed "company for women," hasn't signed. Check the Web site www.safecosmetics.org for updates.

> "The [Food, Drug and Cosmetic Act] contains no provision that requires demonstration to FDA of the safety of ingredients of cosmetic products . . . prior to marketing the product. . . . With the exception of color additives and a few prohibited ingredients, a cosmetic manufacturer may use essentially any raw material as a cosmetic ingredient and market the product without approval from FDA."
>
> —FDA, 2005

WHAT YOU SHOULD KNOW

- The cost of making cosmetics is roughly 20 percent product and 80 percent marketing. Advertising for conventional cosmetics is backed by star endorsements and cultural pressure.

- Modern makeup is largely chemically based and not tested for safety.

- The CIR, or Cosmetic Ingredient Review, panel is in charge of reviewing the safety of cosmetic ingredients in the United States. The Cosmetic, Toiletry and Fragrance Association (recently renamed as the Personal Care Products Council) is the industry's trade association that funds the CIR.

- There hasn't been much research into the safety of nanoparticles in cosmetics. These molecules are so tiny that can go just about anywhere—including, possibly, across the blood–brain barrier. (We'll talk more about this later in the chapter.)

3 WAYS TO MAKE A SHIFT

1. Keep it simple. Buy products with the fewest and safest ingredients possible. Reading labels is essential—and in the case of cosmetics, a magnifying glass may be necessary! (I've seen a bottle of white nail polish with the ingredient list printed on the bottle in white ink. It was impossible to read. One might assume that the manufacturer has something to hide.) As with ingredients on food packaging, labels on cosmetics are written in descending order, so the first ingredients on the list make up the majority of the product. Manufacturers may add certain ingredients to make their products *seem* natural, but if the good stuff appears last on the list instead of first, it means that less than one percent of the product is actually natural, with the rest consisting of chemicals.

2. Do your homework. If you want to know what chemicals are in your cosmetics, visit the Environmental Working Group's online database, listing more than 27,000 products. Log on to www.safecosmetics.org, go to the "Skin Deep Report," and type in the brand name. The Web site also offers a complete list of the cosmetic companies that have pledged to reformulate ingredients to match the EU's guidelines. If your product of choice isn't there, you can enter any suspicious-looking ingredients into the chemical database, called Scorecard, run by the Environmental Defense Fund at www.scorecard.org.

3. Choose trusted companies and safe ingredients. More cosmetic companies are making an effort to offer environmentally friendly products that contain natural and organic ingredients and fewer chemicals and preservatives. When purchasing products, choose from the Great Natural Makeup Lines (see the list on page 84) or look for companies that have signed the Compact for Safe Cosmetics. Go to www.safecosmetics.org to see which companies are on the list.

HOW TO FIND AND CHOOSE SAFE COSMETICS

It's time to take a look at the cosmetic products that you use each day. But before you go and throw away all your current makeup and replace it with natural alternatives, let's understand what "natural" actually means. Since organic beauty and body care products are becoming more popular with consumers (in the United States, sales of natural/organic skin care products, hair care products, and cosmetics rose to $7 billion in 2008), many mainstream

"Natural" and Truly Natural

Though there is no US government regulation of the use of the term *natural* on cosmetics, in May 2008, the National Products Association (NPA)—an industry trade group—announced its own standards for natural product certification. To receive the NPA seal, a product must contain 95 percent truly natural ingredients (meaning ingredients derived from renewable sources found in nature) and may not contain any ingredients with suspected human health risks.

brands are starting to market "natural" products. But just because the label says it's natural doesn't automatically mean a product is healthy or better for the planet, because there are no guidelines in the industry for what constitutes "natural"—or "pure" or "gentle," for that matter. I think it's worth repeating: There is no government agency evaluating these claims, including safety. The beauty industry is self-regulating.

When I checked the selection of "natural" makeup at my local food market and drugstore, the majority contained unpronounceable ingredients, including synthetic chemicals (usually made with petrochemicals), preservatives, artificial colors, fragrances, and parabens. When I checked my health food store, I was surprised to see some of the very same ingredients. Companies are making claims that they use "organic" ingredients, when in fact only one ingredient in 20—such as organic lavender, for example—is truly organic; the rest are synthetic.

Right now, the best way to tell if a product is clean and safe is to see whether it carries the USDA Organic seal (which confirms that at least 95 percent of the ingredients are certified organic, excluding water and salt), the seal from the British Soil Association (the equivalent of the USDA in Europe), or the Natural Products Association (NPA) seal on the label.

You also might want to visit the Web site www.ecofabulous.com. It does research on natural and organic brands and can help you navigate the constantly expanding world of green products. Also check the cosmetic safety database by the Environmental Working Group, Skin Deep, if you have questions about the makeup you are currently using: www.cosmeticsdatabase.com.

GETTING STARTED

OK, ready to make some changes? Pull out all your cosmetics. Since the list of chemicals known to be toxic or contaminated is so long, I've compiled a short "starter list" that's pretty straightforward. (For the complete list, go to the Recommended Resources at the end of the book.) Now, read your labels and put aside any product containing even one of the following ingredients:

- Parabens (methyl-, propyl-, butyl- and ethyl-). They are used as antimicrobial preservatives in more than 13,000 cosmetic products. (I discuss parabens further in chapter 6.)

- Toluene or butylated hydroxytoluene (BHT), which contains toluene. Other names include benzoic and benzyl. Found in lipsticks, sunscreen, blush, shampoo, makeup remover, and concealer.

- Urea (imidazolidinyl) and DMDM hydantoin. These are preservatives that release formaldehyde. Found in moisturizers, mascara, deodorant, douche, body scrubs, and shampoos.

Unlabeled Phthalates

There's another group of chemicals to avoid called phthalates (pronounced THA-lates). In addition to being used to soften items such as plastic toys and vinyl floor tiles, they also keep your mascara from running, stop your nail polish from chipping, and help fragrances linger. Scientists have shown that they are probable human carcinogens as well as endocrine disruptors—

Choosing Cosmetics for the Younger Set

The Environmental Working Group has some suggestions for keeping makeup safe for kids:

1. No powders. Opt for cream-based blushers and eye shadow.

2. Look for phthalate- and toluene-free nail polish.

3. Stick with fragrance-free products.

4. Go easy on the lipstick. Opt instead for a tasty, shiny, beeswax-based lip balm.

5. Use common sense. No playing with eyeliner or mascara, and no cosmetic glitter.

gender-bender chemicals that make girls develop earlier and reduce testosterone levels in boys. One study, from the University of Puerto Rico, reported in the journal *Environmental Health Perspectives* in 2000, found that Puerto Rican girls with premature breast development had high phthalate levels in their blood.

Cosmetics companies insist that the small amounts of phthalates they use are completely harmless. But it's impossible to know how much you're being exposed to because you will never see the word "phthalate" on a label. Phthalates, along with many other chemicals, do not have to be named on product labels because of a loophole in legislation designed to protect the commercial or "trade" secrets of manufacturers.

Ingredients like phthalates are often grouped under the catchphrase "other" or "inert," for example. They could be extremely hazardous to your health. Vinyl chloride used to be considered "inert" and was withheld from labeling until an epidemic of cancers spread through the manufacturing plants using vinyl chloride in the aerosols that were used in beauty parlors in the late 1960s. Also, if you see the word "parfum" on a product label, know that it's another catch-all term synonymous with hidden phthalates.

In 2006, Shanna Swan, PhD, a University of Rochester Professor of environmental medicine and obstetrics/gynecology, released a study in which she collected urine samples from several hundred pregnant women and tested them for nine compounds known to come from metabolizing phthalates. Then she asked pediatricians to conduct a standard genital exam on 134 boys born to these women. She found that boys whose mothers were most exposed to DBP (dibutyl phthalate), an ingredient in nail polish, hair sprays, and perfumes, were more likely to have undescended testicles and smaller penises.

Mercury in the News

In 2008, Minnesota became the first state in the nation to ban intentionally added mercury in cosmetic products. The federal government currently allows a small amount of mercury as a preservative in eye liner, mascara, skin-whitening creams, and freckle creams. "It is known to cause neuro- logical damage in people even in tiny quantities," said Senator John Marty, the Democrat from Minnesota who sponsored the ban. Lawmakers there say they passed the bill with hopes that other states will also do so, forcing the federal government to ban it nationwide.

Types of Phthalates, and Where They Are Found

- DEP (diethyl phthalate): deodorant, fragrance, hair gel, hair mousse, hair spray, hand and body lotions
- DBP (dibutyle phthalate): nail polish, deodorant, fragrance, hair spray
- DEHP (diethylhexyl phthalate): fragrance

Source: Environmental Working Group

No, No Nano

Have you heard about the next new thing in cosmetics and skin care? It's called nanotechnology, in which "unseen," infinitesimally small nanoparticles are being added to cosmetics and body care products. In the medical world they are already being used to successfully deliver drugs across the blood–brain barrier. These microscopically minuscule materials are a billionth of a meter wide, or smaller than a red blood cell and much thinner than a human hair.

Some experts wonder about the risks of these highly engineered nano-structures. There hasn't been much research into their safety. If you apply them to your skin, do they end up in your brain—or, if you're pregnant, in your unborn fetus? Will they do damage? Will other, less welcome, substances piggy-back on them? And what will happen if a number of different nanoparticles, from your face cream, sunscreen, and foundation, join together? We don't know these answers yet. What we do know is that when you mix two or more chemicals together, sometimes you get a substance more powerful than the sum of the individual parts. In other words, 1 + 1 does not equal 2. It can create a chemical reaction packing a powerful punch.

The FDA's Office of Cosmetics and Colors states that it has no nano-specific regulations. In other words, cosmetics manufacturers aren't required to tell the agency if they're using nanotechnology or disclose it on their labels. Here are three *nano* terms you'll be finding in your products.

Nanoemulsians: They're used to encapsulate active ingredients and carry them deeper into the skin.

Nanosomes of pro-retinol A: They penetrate the skin's surface to soften wrinkles and reduce the appearance of fine neck creases.

Nanovectors: They transport and concentrate active ingredients in the skin.

Nanoparticles in Skin Care Products

The following cosmetic companies already are using nanotechnology in some of their products:

Company	Product	Nano-contents
Chanel	Coco Mademoiselle Fresh Moisture Mist	Nanoemulsions
Estée Lauder	Resilience and Renutriv cosmetics	Novasomes
Johnson & Johnson	Neutrogena cosmetics	Novasomes
L'Oreal	Revitalift Double Lifting and Intense Lift Treatment Mask	Nanosomes
Lancôme	Rénergie Microlift	Silicon and protein nanoparticles
Revlon	Colorstay Stay Natural Powder	Aluminium
Christian Dior	DiorSnow Pure UV Base SPF 50	Nano ultraviolet filters

Source: Friends of the Earth

Note that a micronized particle is larger than a nanoparticle, and so is considered to be safe because it doesn't penetrate the skin.

- Micronized particle size = 1 micron = 1,000 nanometers
- Nanoparticle = less than 0.1 micron = 100 nanometers

What's That Smell?

Your favorite department store fragrances are made from chemicals rather than flowers, says Mandy Aftel, natural fragrance guru, and author of *Essence and Alchemy: A Natural History of Perfume*. According to the Environmental

Working Group, there are potentially hundreds of chemicals in a single product's secret fragrance mixture. A number of them are potentially hazardous, including acetone, benzaldehyde, benzyl acetate, benzyl alcohol, camphor, ethanol, ethyl acetate, limonene, linalool, and methylene chloride.

Fragrances are among the top five allergens in the world. Be especially careful with perfumes, since they are applied to the skin repeatedly in concentrated doses. A 2006 Mayo Clinic study placed fragrances (found in cosmetic products, perfumes, and other products) in the 10 most common causes of allergic contact dermatitis, and the Institute of Medicine (a division of the National Academy of Sciences) placed fragrance in the same category as secondhand smoke in triggering asthma in adults and school-age children.

Have you had a whiff of someone wearing a product like a deodorant body spray, for example? I put the words "Avon Naturals Body Spray" into the cosmetics chemical safety database Skin Deep (www.cosmeticsdatabase.com), and four sprays (Banana and Coconut, Cucumber Melon, Tangerine and Aloe, and Sugar Mist) fell into the "highly hazardous" category. They got this score because the ingredients in the products are linked to cancer, neurotoxicity, endocrine disruption, and cellular level changes.

A better choice is to try using perfume, colognes, or body sprays blended from essential oils. Check out these online sources:

- Aftelier Perfumes: www.aftelier.com
- Kate's Magik: www.katesmagik.com
- Natural Perfumers Guild: www.naturalperfumersguild.com (lists members who make fragrances from botanical ingredients)
- Scentual Alchemy: www.scentualalchemy.com

Lead in Lipstick

In October 2007, the Campaign for Safe Cosmetics tested 33 lipsticks and found that one-third contained a "hazardous level" of lead. The cosmetics industry argues that lead is present only in trace amounts. How much lead is OK? Better choose a nontoxic brand!

Great Natural Makeup Lines

The following companies sell makeup that is free of synthetics, parabens, phthalates, petrochemicals, artificial fragrances, and dyes; some are vegan, containing no animal ingredients; and some are organic, containing up to 95 percent certified organic ingredients.

- **Afterglow Cosmetics:** www.afterglowcosmetics.com
- **Aubrey Organics:** www.aubrey-organics.com
- **Cargo:** www.cargocosmetics.com
- **Dr. Hauschka:** www.drhauschka.com
- **Earth's Beauty Cosmetics:** www.earthsbeauty.com
- **Ecobella:** www.ecobella.com
- **Gabriel Cosmetics:** www.gabrielcosmetics.com
- **Jane Iredale:** www.janeiredale.com
- **Lavera:** www.lavera.com
- **Nvey:** www.nveymakeup.com
- **PeaceKeeper:** www.iamapeacekeeper.com
- **Sukicolor:** www.sukicolor.com
- **Weleda:** www.weleda.com

Additional Ways to Make a Shift

- Make your own cosmetics (for sample recipes, see page 87).
- Don't be fooled by brand-name products that say "organic" on the label; read the fine print.
- Choose products that are free of fragrance. Products that claim to be "fragrance free" or "unscented" could contain masking agents that give off a neutral odor. It is best if the word "fragrance" does not appear on the label at all.
- If you use nail polish, make sure you buy a "green" brand at your natural foods market or natural pharmacy. Avoid any brand of polish or polish remover that has toluene or formaldehyde on its label. Even then you should paint your nails in a well-ventilated room.

- After you switch to eco-friendly makeup, replace your makeup brushes with natural ones. (Check out ecoTOOLS, available at drugstores such as Walgreens and Duane Reade.)

Where Else to Shop

Sales of natural and organic cosmetics are soaring, with 2008 marking the beginning of a positive trend. Large department stores such as Macy's, for example, launched a green initiative and slowly introduced "green" cosmetics into their product mix. Target and Walmart began launching their own natural and organic lines. CVS Caremark, the largest U.S. retail pharmacy chain with about 6,300 stores, sent out a news release announcing that it will remove chemicals that have been linked to health problems from its house-branded products and replace them with safer alternatives. This was the first cosmetics safety policy issued by a major drugstore chain in the United States.

Eco-friendly cosmetics are big business at some Sephora stores. Natural and organic products have their own category listing on the company's Web site, www.sephora.com.

Products from Jurlique, an Australian-based natural beauty company, are currently on the shelves of high-end retailers such as Bergdorf Goodman and Barneys New York, and will soon be showing up in more stores across the United States.

Kiehl's, the New York–based skin and hair care company, has been using natural ingredients for about 150 years, ever since the company began as a small apothecary selling tonics and salves to Manhattan locals. They use natural ingredients such as sweet almond oil and yerba maté tea. In 2008 the company began a fair trade initiative with a woman's cooperative in Morocco. You can learn more about their products at www.kiehls.com.

The San Francisco–based beauty giant Bare Escentuals was one of the first cosmetic companies to introduce a mineral-based line of products. Mineral-based products are believed to be better for you because the finely ground minerals are lighter on your skin and don't contain talc, oil, or chemicals.

Cosmetics Without Synthetics, an Arizona-based company, sells more than 500 beauty products from its Web site www.allnaturalcosmetics.com. The most popular lines are Miessence, from Australia, an organic cosmetics and skin care line, and NVEY Eco Organic Makeup, also from Australia.

See the Recommended Resources for more information on healthy, clean cosmetics.

WHAT'S ON THE HORIZON?

We're on the threshold of new possibilities with green chemistry, says Stacy Malkan in her book *Not Just a Pretty Face: The Ugly Side of the Beauty Industry*. "Green chemistry" refers to environmentally friendly chemicals and processes, and the Environmental Protection Agency is supporting the research and development of safer chemicals. Malkan explains that "green chemistry is the recipe for the next industrial revolution, the building block for a new carbon-neutral, toxic-free, zero-waste green economy that lives in harmony with the natural world."

While chemicals in any one product are unlikely to cause harm, here's the bottom line: We are repeatedly exposed to synthetic chemicals from many sources each day. So even a small change, such as switching to a nontoxic lipstick, might make a big difference in your health. If changing up all of your cosmetics feels overwhelming, just start with one thing. Pick your lipstick or

Make Your Own Skin Care Products

It's pretty simple to make your own skin care products from essential oils. These oils are derived from the roots, seeds, leaves, and skins of plants and have been used by many indigenous peoples for thousands of years. Blends of three or more oils are thought by some to create a synergy, yielding a more powerful healing effect on the body. Experiment with different oils. Here are several ways to use them.

- Add two to five drops of essential oils to a basin filled with water; stir. Dip in a clean washcloth, squeeze out the excess water, and apply the cloth to your face.

- Add 20 to 25 drops of one or more essential oils to 2 ounces of sweet almond oil to make a great massage oil.

- Add eight to 10 drops of one or more essential oils in your bath water.

- Add essential oils to simple moisturizing products—10 to 20 drops for every 2 ounces of one of your own unscented, natural moisturizers.

your mascara, whatever. Start with one product a week; by the end of 2 months you'll have a whole new makeup kit!

Recipes

*SKIN-FIRMING BLEND FOR SAGGING SKIN**

8 drops geranium

5 drops helichrysum

2 teaspoons sweet almond oil

5 drops cypress

1 drop peppermint

Add the essential oils to the almond oil and blend well. Massage four to six drops onto the areas where your skin is sagging. Use in the morning and before bedtime.

*ANTI-WRINKLE TREATMENT**

5 drops sandalwood

5 drops helichrysum

5 drops geranium

5 drops lavender

5 drops frankincense

2 tablespoons sweet almond oil

Add the essential oils to the almond oil and blend well. Apply to wrinkle-prone areas. Be careful not to get the oil in your eyes.

UNSUNG HERO

PeaceKeeper Cause-Metics is one of the great natural and organic makeup lines I listed above. Its founder, **Jody R. Weiss**, originally wanted to name her company Revolution Cosmetics because she thought the world needed a revolution in thinking about what real love was, but another company owned the trademark. Then one night she had a dream that her company was called PeaceKeeper. And it wasn't just a cosmetics line; it was a movement.

---

* From the book *Ancient Secrets of Facial Rejuvenation.* Copyright © 2006 by Victoria J. Mogilner. Reprinted with permission of New World Library, Novato, California. www.newworldlibrary.com

3 Things to Look for When Buying Essential Oils

Many essential oils are diluted with other substances, such as carrier oils or even synthetic chemicals. To determine purity, look for these three things:

1. The oil shouldn't leave a greasy residue.

2. The label should state the oil's Latin name, the country of origin, the part of the plant used, and the words "100% pure essential oil."

3. Not all essential oils are priced the same, so if you see a company selling several different oils and each bottle is $9.99, for example, you can be sure that these oils have been diluted or adulterated in some way.

In her dream, Jody saw that women around the world wanted the same thing. The words, in every major language of the world, appeared on the sides of the lipstick carton: freedom, joy, wisdom, voice, esteem. She envisioned borders and flags of nations melting away and women feeding each other's children instead of fighting for food.

Jody left her career as a sports agent in 1996 to devote her time to raising awareness and funds for women's issues. As she explains, "I started PeaceKeeper because I wanted an easy and active way for women to help other women simply by choosing a beauty product." Jody has dedicated her life to promoting peace in the world and in her personal life. Her company makes all-natural and organic lipsticks and lip gloss and eco-safe nail polish, and it is the first cosmetics line to give all of its after-tax distributable profits to women's health and human rights advocacy organizations. PeaceKeeper funds women who live on a dollar a day and those who have been indentured and trains them in a sustainable trade. For more information about the brand and how you can help, go to www.Iamapeacekeeper.com.

Chapter 6

RETHINKING YOUR BODY CARE PRODUCTS

Including Your Soap, Shampoo, Sunscreen, and Toothpaste

"I will buy any creme, cosmetic, or elixir from a woman with a European accent."

—ERMA BOMBECK

AS I'VE BECOME MORE CONSCIOUS of the products I use on my body, I've also made an effort to educate my young daughter about healthy alternatives in soap, shampoo, and toothpaste. In retrospect, my advice might have been a bit severe. When my daughter was about 7 years old, she invited a friend to our home for a sleepover. As they were getting ready for bed, I overheard the following conversation from the bathroom:

Friend: What kind of toothpaste is *that*? It looks weird.

My daughter: It's an all-natural one. And what are you using? Crest? Don't you know that can kill you?

I was horrified. Had I been too harsh in my consciousness-raising and created an eco-monster? I sat them both down and explained that the toothpaste her friend was using wouldn't kill her, or anybody, but that it was better to choose a natural one, without a lot of added chemicals.

We use soap and shampoo to keep our bodies clean, but we may get more than we bargain for each time we use a conventionally made product. In 2005, researchers at the National Institutes of Health discovered that popular shampoos contain a toxic chemical called methylisothiazoline, or MIT, which is linked to nervous system damage. Head & Shoulders, Suave, Clairol products and Pantene Hair Conditioner all contain this ingredient.

As Devra Davis, PhD, points out in her book *The Secret History of the War on Cancer:* "You know how some shampoos leave the hair shiny and smooth? That's because they contain things that bond to the surface of the hair shaft, leaving it silky and under control, but the ways these magical beauty treatments are crafted (in the lab) can be quite unhealthy."

WATCH OUT FOR THESE 3: PHTHALATES, PARABENS, AND DEA

Since most of us buy commercially made body care products produced in a lab, it's important to be aware of the three potentially harmful chemicals found in most of them:

Phthalates: As I mentioned in chapter 5, phthalates are hidden in makeup and perfume, but they also are found in body care products such as deodorant, body wash, baby wipes, baby powders, liquid soap, sunscreen, and skin lotions, referenced on the label merely as "other." People are not exposed to one phthalate at a time. For example, a 2008 research study on baby care products conducted by the Study for Future Families reported that over 80% of all the babies tested had at least seven different phthalates in their urine.

Parabens (alkyl-p-hydroxybenzoates): These chemicals are found in most commercially made soaps and shampoos. The Environmental Protection Agency (EPA) states that all parabens—methyl, propyl, and butyl—are endocrine disruptors, interfering with the function of the endocrine system, which consists of the thyroid, pituitary, adrenal glands, pancreas, and ovaries and testes and which regulates hormones. The Center for Children's Health and the Environment at Mount Sinai School of Medicine in New York City reports that endocrine disruptors have been suspected of contributing to reproductive and developmental disorders, learning problems (such as attention-deficit disorder), and immune system dysfunction. In addition, parabens have been found in breast tumors.

DEA (diethanolamine and its derivatives, cocamide DEA/lauramide DEA and monoethanolamine [MEA]): It's a wetting, thickening, and foaming agent used in shampoos, bath products (including baby wash), liquid hand soaps, shaving products, and deodorants. This group of chemicals has been shown to interfere with normal brain development in baby mice when applied to the skin of pregnant mice, according to researchers at the University of North Carolina at Chapel Hill.

The Cancer Prevention Coalition says that while a product sits on a store shelf or in your cabinet at home, DEA can react with other ingredients in the formula to form an extremely potent carcinogen called nitrosodiethanolamine (NDEA). This is readily absorbed through the skin and has been linked with stomach, esophagus, liver, and bladder cancers. The International Agency for Research on Cancer recommends that NDEA be treated as if it were a carcinogen in humans.

BE CAUTIOUS ABOUT "NATURAL" AND "ORGANIC" PRODUCTS, TOO!

As you now know, most conventionally made personal care products contain nasty chemicals, but some "natural" products do as well. In March 2008, the Organic Consumers Association announced that a cancer-causing compound called 1,4-dioxane has been found in personal care products (and some cosmetics) from top-selling natural and organic manufacturers. The study reported that products from such companies as Kiss My Face, Jason, Citrus Magic, Whole Foods 365, Alba Botanical, Lifetree, Giovanni, and Nature's Gate Organics, among others, contained this carcinogen. It was found mostly in items such as deodorants, shampoos, toothpastes, and mouthwashes.

The discovery that this chemical occurs in top-selling "natural," "organic," or "green" body care products, including those for babies (bubble bath and shampoo), is shocking. And the levels weren't insignificant—they were up to 1,000 times higher than the EPA considers hazardous! When I dug a little deeper into understanding how and why this is possible, I learned that the chemical is not added to products; rather, it is a by-product of a process that softens detergents. It is formed when petrochemicals are used in manufacturing. And here's something else I uncovered, much to my

To avoid the chemical 1,4-dioxane, the Organic Consumer Association (OCA) urges consumers to search ingredient lists for words ending in the letters "eth," such as "myreth," "oleth," "laureth," "ceteareth." Other words to look for include "PEG," "polyethylene," "polyethylene glycol," "polyoxyethylene," or "oxynol."

dismay: So far there are no standards that govern the words "natural" or "organic" for personal care products.

The best way to protect yourself is to choose companies known for their purity and integrity. Also, use a trusted source of information such as the Environmental Working Group (EWG)'s online database of personal care items: www.cosmeticsdatabase.com. It identifies ingredients that may be linked to allergies or cancer.

3 WAYS TO MAKE A SHIFT

1. Read labels and buy products with the fewest and safest ingredients possible (that means no unpronounceable words). By cutting down on the number of chemicals contacting your skin, you will reduce potential health risks associated with your products.

2. Choose products that are free of fragrance. Products that claim to be "fragrance free" or "unscented" could contain masking agents that give off a neutral odor, so it is best if the word "fragrance" does not appear on the label at all.

3. Keep it simple and make your own. (You'll find a few recipes later in this chapter.)

Safe Alternative Ingredients for Skin Care Products

- Coconut oil. Look for a high-quality organic brand that is free of chemicals. The label should say "virgin," "unbleached," and "not hydrogenated."

Making Discerning Choices

CHEC, the Children's Health Environmental Coalition, says don't get tricked by marketing claims used on personal care products because they are not regulated. These include the following terms:

- Hypoallergenic
- Doctor tested
- Doctor approved
- Dermatologist tested or approved
- Nontoxic
- No synthetic ingredients

- Shea butter
- Essential oils
- Kukui nut oil. A good source of this oil, which comes from Hawaii, is http://oilsofaloha.com.
- Organic oils, such as olive, jojoba, sesame, and apricot
- Grapefruit seed extract (used as a preservative). Choose one that is organic and cold pressed (not heated), if possible.

Companies Selling Truly Organic Products

All of the companies listed below sell products found in natural food markets such as Whole Foods, at Beauty Brands and Sephora, and at some conventional pharmacies such as Walgreens and CVS.

- Dr. Bronner's
- EO
- ErbaOrganics
- Miessence (found only online: www.miessenceproducts.com)
- Origins Organics
- Pangea Organics
- PeaceKeeper Cause-Metics
- Queen Helene
- Sun Dog
- TerrEssentials

Companies Selling Products without Harsh, Artificial Ingredients

- Aubrey Organics
- Avalon Organics
- Burt's Bees
- Desert Essence
- Dr. Hauschka
- Ecco Bella
- Honeybee Gardens
- Intellesthetics
- Jurlique
- Liz Earle
- Max Green Alchemy
- MyChelle
- The Organic Make-up Company
- This Works
- Vermont Soapworks
- Weleda
- Yes to Carrots
- Zia Fresh

"Natural" Companies That Sell Products with at Least One Ingredient Deemed Harmful by the EPA

- Alba
- Giovanni
- Jason
- Kiss My Face
- Lifetree

- Method
- Nature's Gate
- Sea-Chi Organics
- Whole Foods 365

TOXIC TOOTHPASTE?

Another way to absorb chemicals in our personal care products is through the mouth. When a drug such as nitroglycerine is administered for a heart condition, it is given under the tongue for fast absorption. So are natural homeopathic remedies. So what happens with your toothpaste? You may be getting a

Reading Labels

When you read product labels, you never know what you'll find. Here's an amazing story from the *New York Times* about a man in Panama who was responsible for setting off a worldwide hunt for tainted toothpaste. Eduardo Arias, who happened to look at a label on a 59-cent tube of toothpaste that he bought at a mall one day, noticed that the label said it contained diethylene glycol, a sweet-tasting, poisonous ingredient in antifreeze that had been mixed into cold syrup in Panama the year before, killing or disabling at least 138 people.

Mr. Arias reported his discovery, and authorities tracked down the tainted toothpaste as coming from China. These small tubes from two well-known brands, Colgate and Sensodyne, had been distributed to prisoners, hospitals, and high-end hotels in the United States. They turned up on six continents, in 34 countries around the world; Japan alone had 20 million tubes.

People had unwittingly been putting an ingredient of antifreeze into their mouths until Mr. Arias spoke up. His alertness and willingness to call attention to what was in the toothpaste forced countries around the world to re-examine how they monitor exports from China and elsewhere.

dose of toxic ingredients during your daily routine of brushing your teeth. Ever look at the warning on your toothpaste box or that of your child's? It says "Keep out of reach of children under the age of six. If more than used for brushing is swallowed, contact the poison control center or your physician."

Look for the USDA or British Soil Association (BSA) Organic Seal on personal care products.

Manufacturers are aware that the chemicals inside the tubes—fluoride, saccharin, additives such as sodium lauryl sulfate (SLS), and antimicrobials such as triclosan and acetylpyridium chloride—should not be ingested in large amounts. But what about small amounts ingested twice a day over years? No one is certain. Plus, triclosan can react with the chlorine in your tap water and turn them into chloroform and dioxins, which are linked to cancer. In other words, if you are brushing your teeth with toothpaste that has triclosan in it, and you are rinsing with tap water that has chlorine in it, you might be getting a little chemical reaction right in your mouth!

EXTREME CLEAN

When it comes to cleaning your skin, don't even think about using antibacterial soaps! According to Johns Hopkins University research, about 75 percent of the bacteria-killing chemical triclosan that people flush down their drains survives treatment at sewage plants, and most of that ends up in sludge spread on farm fields. Every year, the study says, an estimated 200 tons of triclocarban and triclosan (found in antibacterial soaps and toothpaste) are applied to agricultural lands nationwide. Other research from Johns Hopkins suggested that triclocarban was among the top 10 contaminants in waterways. Triclosan, meanwhile, was among the most prevalent in a national analysis of streams by the US Geological Survey.

If you're wondering how you can kill bacteria and keep your hands clean,

MYTH: Antibacterial soaps keep your family healthy and germ-free.
TRUTH: Antibacterial soaps are no more effective than plain soap and water for killing disease-causing germs. And not all "germs" are bad. We need them to maintain healthy immune systems.

an independent federal advisory panel reported that popular antibacterial soaps and washes offer no more protection than regular soap and water. The panel, which advises the FDA, said by an 11-1 vote that it saw no added benefits to antibacterials when compared with soapy hand washing and that soaps that use synthetic chemicals could contribute to the growth of bacteria that are resistant to antibiotics. These antibacterial soaps also dry out your hands, making you lose precious skin oils that are part of your immune system and keep your hands youthful looking!

Super Soaps

Here's a list of some terrific all-natural, earth-friendly soaps made without parabens or petroleum products:

- **DayBreak Lavender Farm:** www.daybreaklavenderfarm.com
- **Herbaria All Natural Soap:** www.herbariasoap.com
- **Hugo Naturals:** www.hugonaturals.com
- **SkinnySkinny:** www.skinnyskinnysoaps.com
- **SumBody:** www.sumbody.com
- **The Soap Fairy:** www.soapfairy.com

Brad Pitt and cosmetics firm Kiehl's have an eco-friendly body wash, called Aloe Vera Biodegradable Liquid Body Cleanser. It contains no parabens, sodium lauryl sulfate, sodium laureth sulfate, or dyes. All profits will benefit JPF Eco Systems, a foundation "supporting global environmental initiatives that minimize impact on the environment." You can buy it at Kiehl's counters in department stores or at: www.kiehls.com

RECONSIDER YOUR SUNSCREEN

When I was a teen living in a New York City suburb, I used to mix baby oil and iodine and rub it on my skin before I went to the beach. It's a miracle I don't have extensive sun damage today! Later on I, like many, used the heavily scented popular brands of sunscreens available on the market. Not until recently did I learn about the unhealthy chemicals in them.

In a 2008 investigation of nearly

1000 name-brand sunscreens, the EWG found that many are not safe and not effective. More precisely, four out of every five contain chemicals that may pose health hazards or don't adequately protect people from UVA radiation. The EWG's investigation determined some of the worst offenders to be leading brands such as Coppertone, Banana Boat, and Neutrogena. These three (along with nearly 600 others) contain an ingredient called oxybenzone, a penetration enhancer, or chemical that helps other chemicals penetrate the skin. Oxybenzone that has been linked to allergies, hormone disruption, and cell damage by the U.S. Centers for Disease Control and Prevention.

New labeling laws are set to go into effect in 2009 that will make reading sunscreen labels easier; a product's UVA rating will be based on a four-star system, while the SPF number relates to the UVB protection. But this won't

Protect Your Kids

Every day children are exposed to an average of 27 personal care product ingredients that have not been found safe for kids, according to a national survey conducted in 2007 by Environmental Working Group. A whopping 77 percent of the ingredients in 1,700 children's products reviewed have not been assessed for safety!

If you have infants, check your baby wipes and baby lotions and find alternative products that are safe (some baby wipes are available with aloe instead of propylene glycol). Cut down on your use of powders, especially baby powder on infants. The FDA warns that powders may cause lung damage if inhaled regularly.

Remember that babies recently treated with infant personal care products such as lotion, shampoo, and powder were more likely to have phthalates in their urine than other babies. This is not good news because phthalate exposure in early childhood has been associated with altered hormones as well as increased allergies, runny nose, and eczema. If you want to decrease your baby's exposure to phthalates, limit the amount of baby care products you use and apply lotions or powders only if it's a medical necessity.

The EWG's investigation found that 1,4-dioxane was found in:

55% of baby bubble baths
57% of baby shampoos
55% of baby soaps

rectify other problems with sunscreen, such as the fact some popular ones break down when exposed to sunlight and some can penetrate the skin, which can contribute to health problems.

Back in the 1970s, Howard Maibach, MD, then a professor in the Department of Dermatology at the University of California, San Francisco, School of Medicine, warned that up to 35 percent of sunscreen applied to the skin passes through and enters the bloodstream. In addition, the longer sunscreen chemicals are left on the skin, the greater the absorption into the body. Frank Garland, PhD, of the University of California, San Diego, has since pointed out that while sunscreens do protect against sunburn, there is no scientific proof that they protect against melanoma or basal cell carcinoma in humans.

Also, many sunscreens on the market use nanotechnology in their formulas. Even if your sunscreen says it has no nano particles in it, don't always believe it; many zinc and titanium sunscreens contain nanosize particles, even when they are not listed on the label.

As you'll recall from the previous chapter, nanoparticles are infinitesimally small, and the scary thing is you don't know how far and how deep they can travel in the body. What if they can cross the blood–brain barrier? Many dermatologists caution their patients about products that contain nanoparticles. Unfortunately, companies don't have to tell you that nanoparticles are in their products, and the EWG has found that more than one-third of all products they tested contain ingredients in nano forms.

Chemicals to Avoid When Purchasing a Sunscreen

- Oxybenzone and dixoybenzone (or 4 MBC)
- PABA (para amino benzoic acid)
- Parabens
- Cinnamates (octyl methoxycinnamate and cinoxate)
- Digalloyl trioleate
- Menthyl anthranilate
- Salicylates (homomenthyl salicylate, octyl salicylate, and triethanolamine salicylate, ethylhexyl salicylate)
- Avobenzone (butyl-methyoxydibenzoylmethane, parsol 1789)

Some "Safer" Sunscreens

In 2008, the sunscreen brand Keys Soap Solar RX Therapeutic Sunblock (in 2007, it was the brand UV Natural) was ranked #1 by the EWG as the safest and most effective sunscreen sold in the United States. Other safe and effective brands include:

- Aveeno Baby
- Badger
- Burt's Bees Chemical Free Sunscreen
- California Baby
- Kabana Green Screen
- Lavera
- Soleo Organics
- Sun Science Sport Formula

These can be purchased at natural foods markets such as Whole Foods and Elephant Pharmacy, at REI, or online at Sun Protection Center (www.SPFstore.com) or at Drugstore.com. Also, check the EWG's Web site for a complete list of safe sunscreen brands (www.cosmeticsdatabase.com), as well as the sunscreen database at www.safecosmetics.org.

Making Your Own

According to clinical nutritionist Krispin Sullivan, CN, author of *Naked at Noon: Understanding Sunlight and Vitamin D*, research shows that a topical application of a 10 percent solution of ascorbic acid (vitamin C) can prevent sun damage to skin. If applied one or more times per day, no sunscreen is necessary. The vitamin C is incorporated into the skin's cells to prevent ultraviolet damage to DNA. It does not wash off. This solution can also be applied after burning to reverse damage already sustained. There are no side effects.

To neutralize chlorine in your bath water, add 1 tablespoon ascorbic acid to the water, says nutritionist Krispin Sullivan.

RECIPES FOR NATURAL SUNSCREEN
SUN SKIN SPRAY

4 ounces distilled water (or 4 ounces George's Aloe Juice, or 4 ounces
Home Health Rose Water)

1 level teaspoon ascorbic acid powder

(Optional: add a few drops of lavender essential oil)

Put in 4-ounce spray bottle. Shake and use one or two times a day before
sunning. Put makeup or other creams or lotions over the top. Always respray
when you have finished sunning.

SUN SKIN LOTION

Use the same recipe as above, but add 1 ounce glycerin (found in any drugstore).
Put in a 4-ounce twist lock pump bottle.

Apply makeup or other creams or lotions over the top. Always respray when
finished sunning. Do not make more than 4 ounces at a time unless you are
using it for your entire body. Vitamin C is readily destroyed in a solution, so it's
best to make a new batch every 5 to 7 days and the lotion every 7 to 10 days.

"This is skin food," says Krispin, "not a topical product." She suggests you
put it on a few hours before going in the sun and let it absorb into the skin.
Also, spray it on after being in the sun to help regenerate the cells. For it to be
most effective, it's important to use pure ascorbic acid, not ester-C or calcium
C or any other derivative.

WHERE TO SHOP

Most often the best personal care products are available in health/natural food
shops, the natural food section of grocery stores, and shops selling environmentally friendly goods. Increasingly, they can be found in mainstream stores
such as Walmart, Target, and some pharmacies. Many can be ordered online.
One great online source is www.TheBodyDeli.com, which offers "Fresh Food
for the Skin." Most of their body lotions and oils have to be refrigerated to
retain their potency.

Unless our concern grows for what we're putting on our skin, truly natural
products won't have a fighting chance to survive in the market. It's important to
support products from trusted cosmetic and body care companies that use natural,

certified organic, nontoxic, and non-synthetic ingredients. Commit to switching to at least one healthy body care product before you move on to the next chapter. You'll be glad you did!

For the latest updates on truly natural cosmetics and body care products, visit www. supernaturalhome.com.

UNSUNG HERO

Lisa Levin, founder and CEO of Pharmacopia, started her natural and organic body care company because of her own health problems. She had been a stressed-out graphic designer for 20 years when she was diagnosed with fibromyalgia. She was in a lot of pain, her memory was bad, and she was having trouble sleeping, so she took time off from work to take care of herself. She started eating fewer processed foods and using natural products on her body; soon she noticed that she was feeling better. She also studied aromatherapy and herbal medicine, and became intrigued by the healing qualities of plants. "When I saw that there were very few brands that really capitalized on these therapeutic powers, I started to mix my own products and then design bottles for all of the things that I was making. I'd take samples to my friends and they loved my formulas," said Lisa.

Her products are the first organic brand to be sold at Beauty Brands stores, a major retail chain throughout the United States. The product line is vegan and includes therapeutic bath salts, body lotions, hand creams, soaps, lip balms, and shower gels, in four herbal blends of rosemary, ginger, citrus, and lavender; they also have organic soy candles. To check out their products, visit the company Web site: www.pharmacopia.com.

Environmental Impact of Sunscreens

A team of researchers at the European Commission discovered that sunscreen ingredients that wash off swimmers are bleaching coral reefs worldwide. The study, published in the journal *Environmental Health Perspectives*, showed that reefs are being threatened by the 4,000 to 6,000 metric tons of sunscreen that annually wash off swimmers.

In addition, a group of Swiss agriculture department chemists discovered traces of commonly used ultraviolet filters found in sunscreens in the fish in mountain lakes and rivers.

What Surrounds You

How to Minimize Indoor Air Pollution in Your Home Environment

"Remember when atmospheric contaminants were romantically called stardust?"

—LANE OLINGHOUSE

WHEN I WAS ABOUT 14 YEARS OLD, I had my first environmental wake-up call. At sleep-away camp that summer, the kids and staff left the cabins and headed down to the lake while I stayed behind; I wasn't feeling up to the swimming Olympics planned for that day. About an hour later, a truck sprayed the cabins with a thick white fog to rid the area of mosquitoes. I was terrified. I grabbed my pillow, threw myself down on the floor, and buried my face. I was nauseous, my eyes watered, and my throat burned. This frightening experience got my attention. I knew it would somehow be significant in my life.

My second attention-getting event came just a few years ago in the form of another pesticide shower. This time, on a South African Airways flight to Johannesburg, an announcement was made that an "air freshener" would be sprayed in the cabin. An attendant then walked down the aisle, aiming two cans, one to the right and one to the left, spraying an offensively sweet-smelling mist towards the narrow space between the overhead bins and the passengers' heads. All the while, we were required to keep our seatbelts fastened. Again, I buried my face in my pillow. I felt nauseous and dizzy, and I got a headache that lasted for about 2 hours.

I was disgusted that this was done without my permission. I looked around. No one—not even the woman nursing an infant in front of me—was protesting or seemed at all disturbed by the spraying. Was it my past experience that sensitized me to this insult to my senses?

I asked to speak to the head flight attendant, who told me that the spray was to "freshen" the cabin as well as to prevent hoof and mouth disease, and that the World Health Organization said it was "necessary and safe." I asked to see the can and wrote down the name of the active ingredient: permethrin. When I got home and did some research, I discovered that permethrin is found in household insect sprays and in fitted carpets (added by manufacturers to kill dust mites). It's also a neurotoxin. (It is banned for use in aircraft cabins in the United States because of safety concerns, according to the Association of Flight Attendants.)

Now, these dramatic scenarios are not what most people usually have to endure. Still, we are showered with toxic inhalants on a much more subtle yet just as powerful level right where we live. Inside your home you are being exposed to more severe pollution than you'll get from landfills, hazardous waste sites, or smokestacks, say many scientists, including some Environmental Protection Agency (EPA) officials. That's right: Your indoor environment could be more toxic than your outdoor one—even if you live in a highly polluted city such as Los Angeles. Airborne chemicals and dangerous electromagnetic fields are embedded in our daily lives, swirling together while we're talking on our cell phones, painting and papering our walls, cooking in our nonstick pans, and eating off our ceramic dishes. We're dragging them into our homes on our shoes and then stirring them up when we walk on our carpets. They are in the poorly labeled bottles of brightly colored cleaning fluids in our kitchens and bathrooms, and in the bug sprays and air fresheners we use throughout our homes.

Airborne chemicals are actually toxic gases known as VOCs, or volatile organic compounds. These chemicals are deemed volatile because they evaporate into the air and then you breathe them in. They're emitted from things such as paints, air fresheners, new carpets, and plastic shower curtain liners.

VOCs affect all of us—even unborn babies. In 2005 the Environmental Working Group (EWG) commissioned a study of 10 Americans to find out if any toxic chemicals were in their bodies. The analysis detected 287 industrial chemicals. These 10 people weren't adults; they were *newborns!*

The Human Toxome Project, a comprehensive study begun in 2000 by the EWG to analyze human tissues for industrial chemicals, demonstrated this as well when it found chemicals in umbilical cord blood and breast milk. It's clear that wombs are not safe havens from chemicals such as insecticides, pesticides, and heavy metals—some of the worst and most health-damaging toxins around.

Then, as children grow, they crawl and play on floors and carpets, where they are exposed to floor dust that may contain lead and tracked-in chemicals such as pesticides that may harm brain development. It has been suggested that by the time a baby is 6 months old, it has already absorbed about 30 percent of its total lifetime toxic load of chemicals. Today's children harbor way more toxins than their grandparents.

Airborne chemicals also show up in our homes as PBDEs (polybrominated diphenyl ethers), a flame retardant used frequently in furniture foam and on fabrics. They have been shown to accumulate in the blood and breast milk of humans. The technology to test for these flame retardants, known as "body burden" testing, is about 10 years old, but many countries have heeded the warning signs they've seen in animal studies. Sweden banned PBDEs in 1998, and the European Union banned most PBDEs in 2004. Americans have levels of flame retardants in their bodies that are approximately 10 times higher than those of Europeans or Japanese, and levels are doubling every 2 to 5 years, according to the EPA. This could be because the European Union's manufacturing standards are stricter about banning certain toxic chemicals.

The EU has a program called REACH (Regulation on Registration, Evaluation, Authorization and Restriction of Chemicals) that requires industry to prove the safety of their chemicals and consumer products *before* they reach the market. In the United States, the manufacturer of two kinds of PBDEs voluntarily stopped making them in 2004, but a third kind, deca, is still used here in mattresses and textiles.

In 2008, the EWG found that PBDEs, including deca, are polluting the blood of toddlers and preschoolers in levels three times higher than their moms. Scientists believe that they may be absorbing the chemical into their systems in such large amounts because they are touching their environment and then putting their hands in their mouths much more often than adults.

Our bodies are remarkably resilient in defending against the effects of these chemicals, but only to a point. Scientists question the cumulative effect. It is common sense to believe that the more chemicals you are exposed to, the more likely you will eventually be negatively affected by them.

In the next several chapters, we will take a look at several rooms in your home and I will show you simple steps to reduce your contact with harmful chemicals, plus offer safe alternatives.

Chapter 7

THE BEDROOM

How to Improve One of the Most Important Rooms in Your Home

"Life is something that happens when you can't get to sleep."

—Fran Lebowitz

IF YOU HAD TO CHOOSE just one room in your home to eliminate toxic chemicals, it's the bedroom (including the nursery and kid's room). Transforming your bedroom into a healthy and comfortable retreat can have a major impact on improving your health and well-being. Most of us don't give our bedrooms a second thought except to make sure we have a comfortable bed or one that fits with our decor. New parents often make the mistake of buying new furniture, installing new carpeting, and painting the nursery, unknowingly creating a toxic environment for their babies, who are most susceptible to chemical exposures.

The good news is creating a healthy bedroom is pretty simple. Let's start by looking at the most important piece of furniture in the room.

THE BED

You spend about one-third of your life in bed. That's about 25 years with your face pressed up against the materials you sleep on. Mattresses made with synthetic ingredients off-gas, or release chemicals into the air, which you inhale while you are sleeping. Therefore, it's critical that what you're inhaling isn't toxic.

Start by getting a good-quality, natural mattress. The one you're sleeping on right now probably contains polyurethane (PU) foam, Styrofoam, and polyester, which are derived from things such as crude oil and natural gas. PU foam, in particular, degrades over time, causing the mattress to sag and form body impressions. Your mattress has also probably been treated with flame retardants (polybrominated diphenyl ethers, or PBDEs) and water- and stain-resistant chemicals that are recognized carcinogens.

A 2000 medical study from New Zealand attributed crib deaths to off-gassing of chemicals in baby mattresses.

Here are the main chemicals being used by mattress manufacturers to meet current state and federal flammability standards:

- Boric acid
- Antimony trioxide
- Vinylidiene chloride
- Zinc borate

- Melamine
- Formaldehyde
- Decabromodiphenyl oxide
- PBDEs

There can be as much as one and a half pounds of these chemicals in the surface of a queen mattress. Imagine breathing this stuff in every night! No other type of chemical exposure comes close to the intensity and duration of exposure to a mattress. It's in your face, with full body contact, every day, for years.

Mary Cordaro, healthy home specialist and certified Bau-biologist (see Glossary page 205), concurs. She recommends mattresses and bed systems made with high-quality, organic wool batting because organic wool is naturally fire retardant and dust mite resistant, wicks and dries moisture away from the body, and cushions the body. "Since the average body loses about a pint of vapor into the bed every night, it's important that the battings used in beds and bedding efficiently and effectively wick and dry, so that conditions favorable for mold and dust mites are eliminated," Cordaro says.

3 WAYS TO MAKE A SHIFT

1. Sleep on a mattress made from untreated, nontoxic natural materials containing no synthetic chemicals or fire retardants.

2. If you can't afford a new mattress, buy a wool and organic cotton mattress topper.

3. Buy a solid wooden bed instead of one made of particleboard or fiberboard, which can give off toxic fumes. (See chapter 8 for more information on wood furniture.)

Where to Shop

There are a variety of organic and green mattresses on the market at a variety of prices. The Simmons Natural Care by Danny Seo is sold at JCPenney. These mattresses are made with a natural latex top and are resistant to dust mites, mold, and mildew. A soy-base foam (made from renewable soybeans) lies beneath the latex to add support. The outer layer of fabric is made from Tencel, a biodegradable material made from cellulose. The mattresses are treated not with PBDE but rather with a nontoxic salt-based fire retardant. The wood used in the frame is from accredited and sustainably managed forests, while the steel is made from at least 80 percent recycled materials.

Stores such as European Sleepworks offer moderately priced all-natural mattresses; Duxiana, Shifman, and Mcroskey are on the high end. Then there's Hastens, with probably the most expensive bed on the planet: A top-of-the-line, hand-crafted bed can cost between $18,000 and $60,000 (although their entry-level model is about $4,000). If you're looking for a nontoxic but inexpensive mattress, check out IKEA, which prohibits the use of brominated flame retardants in all their furniture and mattresses, although here in the United States it treats mattresses with organic phosphor or nitrogen-based flame retardants.

There are no standard labels on mattresses listing flame retardant chemicals, so it's important to check with the manufacturer or store before purchasing. Inventory changes, so there could be new lines that are now flame-retardant free. Remember that if you can't afford to buy a new mattress, you can get a mattress topper made from organic cotton and wool. Or use a mattress cover made from barrier cloth. This tightly woven fabric has a thread count of 300 or higher to help isolate an unhealthy mattress.

The following Web sites offer organic mattresses and bedding:

- **Anna Sova:** www.annasova.com (organic sheets and towels, too)
- **E3 Environmental:** www.h3environmental.com (Mary Cordaro's Web site)

- **Earthsake:** www.earthsake.com
- **Good Night Naturals:** www.goodnightnaturals.com
- **Holy Lamb Organics:** www.holylamborganics.com
- **Keetsa mattresses:** www.keetsa.com
- **Lifekind:** www.lifekind.com
- **Natura Bed Systems:** www.nontoxic.com/natura
- **The Natural Mattress Store:** www.thenaturalmattressstore.com
- **Nirvana Safe Haven:** www.nontoxic.com
- **Shepherds Dream:** www.shepherdsdream.com
- **Soaring Heart:** www.soaringheart.com

For healthy baby mattresses and bedding:

- **Criblife2000:** www.criblife2000.com (information on creating a safe and healthy sleeping environment for babies)
- **Dax Stores:** www.daxstores.com
- **Green Nest:** www.greennest.com
- **Tiny Birds Organic Baby:** www.tinybirdsorganics.com

Mattress Law

Hundreds of people die each year in house fires that begin when someone falls asleep with a cigarette in hand, igniting a mattress. Beginning in 2007, mattresses made and sold in the United States are required to meet tough new federal standards, proving they can withstand a blast of fire without bursting into flames. To meet this standard, new mattresses use a barrier system just under the ticking that is filled with toxic flame-retardant chemicals. One of these chemicals is antimony trioxide, which the CPSC (Consumer Product Safety Commission) calls a "probable carcinogen." Many mattresses use boric acid, or common household roach killer, to meet the flammable standard. In the United States, you currently need a doctor's note to buy a boric acid–free mattress.

Feng Shui in the Bedroom

Almost as important as *what* your bed is made of is *where* it is placed in your bedroom. According to the principles of the ancient art known as feng shui (pronounced *fung shway*), the placement of furniture in your home can affect your health, wealth, personal relationships, and overall well-being.

I remember when my husband and I bought the home we now live in. To me, something seemed "off" about the master bedroom. The position of the closet forced the bed to be placed facing the bathroom, with the toilet in plain sight. I intuitively thought this wasn't a good thing.

I once read that the view from your bed influences the way you view your life, since it's the first thing you see in the morning and the last thing you see at night. Fortunately, before we moved in, we were able to have a carpenter reposition the door to the closet so that the bed could fit along a wall that faced a large window. I now wake up every morning grateful for the opportunity to look at sky and trees, instead of the toilet. Waking up grateful sets a positive tone for my day, which is a good thing.

According to some feng shui practitioners, if you want to get a good night's sleep, it's important that your body feels safe and you have a deep sense of inner security. Otherwise you can remain tense while you're asleep, and you may wake up fatigued or with a stiff neck!

According to feng shui principles, here are suggestions for optimal bed placement:

- Position your bed so that you can see the door from where you sleep, without being directly in front of the door.

- If your bed must be in front of the door, put a substantial footboard, trunk, table, or seat at the foot of the bed.

- Allow one side of the bed to touch a wall.

- Place the headboard slightly away from the wall.

- Make sure the space under the bed is free from clutter.

Another ancient Asian system of architecture and sacred space is called vastu. It is a spiritual, scientific design system from India's Vedic tradition and is called "the Yoga of design." For more information: www.transcendencedesign.com or www.kaleshwaravaastu.com

Sheets, Blankets, Pillows, and Pillow Cases

I don't know about you, but I love the feel of getting between two freshly laundered sheets. I used to buy what looked pretty and felt soft. I sought out designer sheets, which usually were a blend of cotton and polyester. Then I discovered that all cotton/polyester blend permanent press ("easy care," "no iron") fabrics have formaldehyde finishes that cannot be washed out.

I also looked for "Egyptian cotton" sheets, since the fabric is synonymous with luxury and renowned for its wonderful texture. As I learned, however, much of the cotton is picked or processed by children, some as young as 5 or 6. The British charity Environmental Justice Foundation, which has investigated the cotton industry around the world, points out that Egyptian cotton's production is linked with child labor—up to 1 million children are working in Egyptian cotton fields every year. So, it's important to choose organic or fair trade brands to be sure that no child labor was involved.

3 WAYS TO MAKE A SHIFT

1. Choose 100 percent cotton sheets. If you want the best, choose *organic* cotton. Even if the label on a conventional cotton sheet says it's all natural, undyed, and unbleached, such claims don't guarantee that the cotton was grown and manufactured without toxic chemicals.

2. Try bamboo sheets. They feel incredibly soft and are very affordably priced. Most bamboo is processed using strong chemical solvents that are linked to health problems; the difference is that the chemicals aren't permanently embedded in the fabric. This is why bamboo manufacturers can claim that their products are "chemical-free." Look for the Fair Trade Federation label or the Co-op America's Business Seal of Approval, to be safe.

3. If you like wool blankets, try to find "Pure Grow Wool" or "Eco Wool" that hasn't been treated with toxic mothproofing pesticides. Wool fibers absorb and store moisture, and also trap pockets of air that regulate temperature in every season and climate. Wool is a naturally hypoallergenic product that is resistant to dust mites, mold, and mildew.

The Benefits of Organic Cotton

Cotton needs huge amounts of water and lots of chemicals to grow. It is one of the most intensively sprayed field crops in the world. The USDA reports that more than 53 million pounds of pesticides and 1.6 billion pounds of synthetic fertilizers are applied to cotton fields annually. Organic cotton, on the other hand, is grown without chemical agents (fields must be free of synthetic chemicals for 3 years before they are certified). Plus, many organic cotton products are free of synthetic dyes.

Where to Shop

Department stores are starting to stock organic sheets and towels. Macy's now offers a home line that uses natural fibers and low-impact dyes. Haven by Hotel Collection, Macy's private home brand, features 100 percent organic sheets and throws. I also found some organic sheets and towels at Bed Bath & Beyond; a certified organic cotton collection at West Elm (www.westelm.com); and a kids' line of organic cotton sheets and blankets at Pottery Barn (www.pbteen.com).

For pillows, check out:

- **EcoBedroom:** www.ecobedroom.com
- **Rawganique:** www.rawganique.com
- **Serenity Pillows:** www.serenitypillows.com (ergonomic pillows made from organic buckwheat or millet hulls and eco-wool)

DUST MITES

Dust mites are microscopic creatures that live by the millions in mattresses and bedding (and in couches, carpet, stuffed toys, and old clothing, too!). They were first discovered in 1694 by the inventor of the microscope, Anton van Leeuwenhoek. Dust mites feed on the dead skin that sloughs off our bodies (as well as our pets'). They are second only to pollen in causing allergic reactions. If you suspect you are allergic to them, follow these guidelines from the National Institute of Environmental Health Sciences:

- Use a dehumidifier or an air conditioner to maintain relative humidity at about 50% or below.

- Encase your mattress and pillows in dust-proof or allergen-impermeable covers (available online and at some department stores).

- Wash all bedding and blankets once a week in hot water (at least 130°F). Nonwashable bedding can be frozen overnight to kill dust mites. Use perfume-free, biodegradable detergents when washing your sheets.

- If possible, replace wall-to-wall carpets with bare floors (linoleum, tile, or wood) and remove fabric curtains and upholstered furniture.

- Vacuum often with a vacuum cleaner equipped with a high-efficiency particulate air (HEPA) filtration system. Throw away vacuum bags after use because dust mites can leave the bag.

- Wear a mask while vacuuming to avoid inhaling allergens, and stay out of the vacuumed area for 20 minutes after cleaning to allow any dust and allergens to settle.

LOSING SLEEP OVER EMFs

Since we spend so much time in the bedroom, it's important to consider how electricity might be polluting it. Our bedrooms are filled with electrical wiring, and many of us have appliances, such as electric clock radios, televisions, VCRs, telephone answering machines, and computers, near us while we sleep that give off electromagnetic field (EMF) radiation.

Moth Balls

Moth balls are made with pesticides called naphthalene or paradichlorobenzene (PDB), which are considered toxic and possible carcinogens by the Environmental Protection Agency and now banned by the European Union (EU). Instead of moth balls, store your woolens in cedar closets or chests, or use cedar shavings or blocks. Moths are also repelled by cloves, eucalyptus, lavender, cinnamon sticks, and bay leaves. Place in cheesecloth bags and stick in pockets or dangle from hangers. Smells better too! Look for other nontoxic moth ball alternatives at www.care2.com.

Bedroom Wall Color

The color of your walls can affect how you feel in a room. Terah Kathryn Collins, author of *Home Design with Feng Shui*, says the best bedroom colors are the skin colors found in all the races of people around the world. These include creamy beiges and browns, pinks, yellows, and reds; as well as the deeper tones of chocolate, coral, raspberry, butter cream, lavender, burgundy, and aubergine. Pure white, black, gray, blue, and cool greens can be included but will make the bedroom chilly and less inviting if they dominate.

When we are continually exposed to EMFs, they can have a negative effect on our health. In 1990, David Carpenter, MD, then dean of the School of Public Health at the State University of New York, reported that up to 30 percent of all childhood cancers may be due to exposure to residential power lines. In a follow-up study in 2007, Dr. Carpenter, now director of the Institute for Health and the Environment at the University of Albany, asserts that exposure to some kinds of EMF may cause serious health effects, including cancer and neurologic disease. Researchers in Sweden found that adults who are exposed to high magnetic fields at home and at work are 3.7 times more likely to develop leukemia than those who are not. Researchers from Oxford University in the United Kingdom report that children living near high-voltage power lines are substantially more likely to develop leukemia.

Sleeping near a lot of electrical fields can keep you from sleeping soundly. Exposure to elevated levels of electricity, especially at night, can cause headaches, nightmares, depression, and fatigue, as well as long-term illness.

I bought a device known as a Gauss meter (found online, starting at about $35), a hand-held device that measures EMFs in my home. I discovered that there was an extremely high EMF reading directly behind the headboard in the bedroom of another home we were about to buy. A skilled EMF electrician determined that the wall was wired improperly and inexpensively remedied the situation for us.

Do you sleep with an electric blanket? They are known to create a strong magnetic field, and studies have linked them to miscarriages and childhood leukemia. It's been recommended that if you use one don't sleep with it turned on; use it to warm up your bed and shut it off when you climb in.

Electric clocks emit a high magnetic field up to 3 feet away. If you have a bedside clock, it may be wise to place ir at least 2 to 3 feet from where you sleep.

3 WAYS TO MAKE A SHIFT

1. Simplify your sleep space. Try not to have your office in your bedroom.

2. Place all electrical equipment, including your clock, as far away from the head of your bed as possible, because electrical currents may interfere with sleep.

3. Use green plants in the room to help absorb electromagnetic fields. (See Chapter 8 on the best plants to use to purify the air.)

TOXIC TOYS

Toys can be a source of toxicity in kids' rooms and nurseries. Despite all we know about the dangers of lead and other toxic chemicals, the U.S. government doesn't require full testing of chemicals before they are added to toys. So it's not surprising that lead is found in a significant percentage of toys currently on the market. A nonprofit organization called HealthyToys.org decided to take action. They released a report based on research conducted by environmental health organizations and other researchers around the country, which tested over 1,200 children's products. They found lead in 35 percent of these products, with levels in 17 percent exceeding 600 parts per million (ppm). By comparison, the American Academy of Pediatrics (AAP) recommends a level of just 40 ppm as the maximum amount of lead that should be allowed in children's products!

In addition to lead, most kids' toys are made from plastic containing PVC, phthalates, and bisphenol-A (BPA). (Be aware that the rubber duckie, the little yellow bath toy, isn't rubber, but plastic.) For alternatives to plastic, look for toys made of solid wood with nontoxic paints and finishes. It's best to use all-natural fibers such as cotton, hemp, and wool; organic would be the best choice. If it's impossible to do without plastic toys, some companies are now labeling their products "PVC free," so look for that on the package.

Every natural toy you buy makes a difference. It decreases your child's overall exposure to pollutants and can help create demand for natural products in the marketplace. Natural toys can be both beautiful and fun. For example, my daughter enjoys using modeling beeswax. When she holds the wax in her hands it begins to soften. For years, ever since she was in first grade, she has been making the most wonderfully colorful and whimsical creatures, and she hasn't tired of this creative process the way she tired of the plastic dolls she's collected over the years.

California, Washington, and Vermont have banned the use some phthalates in toys (as have Japan and the European Union). About 30 states are considering new regulations on chemicals in toys.

Where to Shop

Toys R Us has come out with a line of natural-wood, paint-free toys, including cars, trucks and blocks.

Green Toys (www.greentoys.com) manufactures toys that are made from recycled curbside collected plastic milk containers and contain no phthalates or BPA. Plus, they have no external coatings—eliminating the fear of lead.

A number of other retailers are selling natural toys, including these:

- **Earthentree:** www.earthentree.com
- **EcoBaby Organics:** www.ecobaby.com
- **Hazelnut Kids:** www.hazelnutkids.com
- **Holgate Toys:** www.holgatetoy.com (wooden, made in the United States)
- **I Love My Planet Toys:** www.ilovemyplanettoys.com
- **Lego:** www.lego.com (phthalate free)
- **Natural Baby Catalog:** http://naturalbabystores.yahoo.net
- **North Star Toys:** www.northstartoys.com
- **Oompa Toys:** www.oompa.com
- **Organic Gift Shop:** www.organicgiftshop.com
- **Peapods Natural Toys:** www.peapods.com
- **Turner Toys:** www.turnertoys.com

DREAM, DREAM, DREAM

Don't forget the magical side of sleep. When your bed is comfortable, it's easier to fall and stay asleep. Getting good-quality sleep allows you to stay healthy and fight off illness because sleep is the time when your body heals, repairs, and rejuvenates. Deep sleep also allows us to dream. When my husband and I moved to California from New York City, we needed a new bed, so we bought a Duxiana. My very first night on it, I had my best night's sleep in years (maybe it was because we had left Manhattan?). I had vivid dreams and awoke refreshed. It's been like that ever since.

UNSUNG HERO

Christi Graham is one of the most passionate and visionary leaders and pioneers in the green building movement today. She is part of a new architectural revolution—bringing aesthetic, environmental, and health interests together into one integrated design.

Christi has spent the past 15 years producing and directing numerous green and healthy living events and programs, and founding non-profit organizations such as the Green Resource Center of Berkeley, California, and the Green Materials Showcase, which has become the largest annual green building trade show on the West Coast. Christi is also the founder and executive producer of West Coast Green, the largest interactive conference and expo in the nation on green innovation, building, and technology; founder and president of Healthy Home Plans, a source for healthy and sustainable home plans designed by award-winning architects; and co-author, editor, and producer of *Healthy Construction Guidelines*, a step-by-step guide to building or remodeling a safe, healthy, and nontoxic home.

Christi's commitment is to revolutionize the way people build and live in their homes, by realigning with the natural world. "By extending the definition of green building beyond the walls of the house and revealing the vital links between the built environment, our total well-being physically, emotionally, and spiritually, and the realization of our true nature as humans, I hope to cast our home and lifestyle choices in an evolutionary light, stirring our deepest appetite for positive change," said Christi.

For more information: www.westcoastgreen.com.

Chapter 8

THE LIVING ROOM, DEN, AND HOME OFFICE

Choosing Safe Flooring, Wall Coverings, and Furniture

"There's so much plastic in this culture that vinyl leopard skin is becoming an endangered synthetic."

—LILY TOMLIN

YOU NEVER REALLY THINK that living in your home could make you tired, irritable, or even sick, but over time your body may absorb a number of potentially toxic substances hiding there. These include common volatile organic compounds (VOCs) such as formaldehyde, emitted by things such as paint and furniture; PBDEs (polybrominated diphenyl ethers), used as flame retardants on fabrics and mattresses; and phthalates, found in things such as plastics, wood, textiles, glues, and sealants.

These chemicals may exacerbate allergies and asthma, and can cause nausea; dizziness; eye, nose and throat irritation; cough; headache; flu-like symptoms; and skin irritation. As they accumulate in the body over time they can silently affect how efficiently your body runs—whether you can maintain a healthy metabolism, burn fat well, and keep your hormones in balance. Some are also known to cause heart, lung, or kidney damage and even cancer and nerve damage if exposure is prolonged. This in turn can have a devastating

No Safety Testing

"It may shock you to learn that of the 100,000 chemicals that are commonly used in commerce, most have not been studied as to their ability to affect our health," says Devra Davis, PhD, author of *The Secret History of the War on Cancer.* The National Academy of Sciences confirmed that we have no public record of the toxicity of three out of four of the top 3,000 chemicals in use today.

effect on your health. If your liver, for instance, becomes taxed by an overburden of chemicals, it may not work efficiently, setting you up for other health problems.

Literally millions of chemicals have been invented by humans in the past 60 years; depending on whom you ask, somewhere between 80,000 and 100,000 are in common use today. Yet only a very tiny percentage have ever been directly tested for their effects on humans, and only a fraction of those tested are building materials.

Here in America, we are being exposed to some products that are restricted by the European Union (EU). The EU is following what's known as the "precautionary principle," where the burden of proof that a product is potentially harmful lies with the chemical companies, not the public. The EU restricts hundreds of chemicals and requires the industry to test most chemicals before they are sold on the market. That's not the case in the United States. Essentially, the only way we know something is toxic is to discover that, after it has been used for years, it has caused problems for thousands of people. This is, of course, why the precautionary principle is so important. If the health effects of a product are unknown, it's best to avoid it whenever possible. In other words, better safe than sorry. With all the untested chemicals in use today, if you don't follow this advice, you just became a test mouse in the study!

Indoor air pollution may be up to 100 times higher than outdoor air pollution, says the Environmental Protection Agency (EPA). Creating an environment free of toxins may seem impossible, but it's not. You may not be able to build a new home using all natural materials, but you can make small changes to bring more natural and healthy materials into your living space. Let's discover how you're exposed and then do a walk-through of your home, where you can make some easy shifts towards "green," less toxic products.

4 Ways You Are Exposed to Indoor Air Pollution in Your Living Room, Den, and Home Office

1. Carpeting and floors
2. Walls
3. Furniture
4. Radiation from cell phones

CARPETING

If you chose carpeting as floor covering, it's important to know that adhesives and other chemicals create fumes that can cause headaches, runny eyes and nose, and odors that can last for years. Many carpets are treated with "stain-resistant" chemicals called telomers, a cousin of Teflon. When you vacuum a carpet that is stain-resistant, the telomers can be released into the air and then breathed in.

New carpets contain the dreaded VOCs that I spoke about in chapter 7. That "new carpet smell" comes from chemicals used in the latex backing. These include toluene, benzene, formaldehyde, ethyl benzene, styrene, acetone, and other chemicals that have made the EPA's list of extremely hazardous substances. New carpets also contain adhesives, stain protectors, and mothproofing that can negatively affect your health. In addition, many new carpets are sprayed with flame retardants. Research has shown that when carpets were analyzed in a lab, they contained high concentrations of heavy metals, such as lead, cadmium, and mercury, PAHs (polycyclic aromatic hydrocarbons), pesticides, and PCBs (polychlorinated biphenols).

Safe Carpet Deodorizer

Debra Lynn Dadd, author of *Home Safe Home*, recommends deodorizing your carpet by sprinkling baking soda liberally over the entire surface (make sure the carpet is dry first). "By 'liberally,' I mean it should look as if it had snowed on the carpet," says Dadd. "You will need several pounds for a 9 by 12 foot room. Wait 15 minutes or longer, then vacuum." Dadd tried it with an old wool Oriental area rug that was musty from sitting in an attic; after two applications, the odor was completely gone.

Old carpets can be just as hazardous. They not only contain the chemicals banned from more recent production, they also have had years to accumulate dust mites, dirt, pesticides, and other toxins brought in on shoes and pets' paws. Did you know that your carpet can hold eight times its weight in toxin-filled dirt? If the carpet is plush or shag, there's probably more dirt hiding in it.

If you want to remove a carpet from the floor, it's best to have a professional pull it up so it doesn't kick up particles into the air. If you will be removing carpeting yourself, Mary Cordaro, the healthy home specialist mentioned in chapter 7, recommends sealing off the room from the rest of the house, sealing all heating/air conditioning registers in the room, bagging and sealing the carpet and removing it from the room, and then hiring a mold abatement company to deep-clean the room.

3 WAYS TO MAKE A SHIFT

1. If you must buy a new carpet, choose one made of wool. It's naturally flame retardant, nontoxic, and nonallergenic, and it deters bacterial growth. Also, the moisture content of wool reduces static electricity. Don't glue your new carpet to the floor; instead, attach it with tackless strips around the room's perimeter and staple it to the subfloor. Be sure to use untreated carpet pads, too.

2. Vacuum with a well-sealed, high-quality high-efficiency particulate air (HEPA) vacuum cleaner. This can do a much better job of cleaning your carpets than the cheaper vacuum cleaners found at most department stores. Steam cleaning can kill dust mites and bacteria.

3. A good doormat will stop a lot of toxins right at the door. Or, take your shoes off when entering your house.

Where to Shop

- **Earthweave:** www.earthweave.com (Bio-Floor wool area rugs containing no dyes or stain-resisting treatments; the adhesives are natural rubber with jute backing)

- **Flokati:** www.flokatirug.net (100% wool area rugs that are handmade in Greece)

- **Rawganique:** www.rawganique.com (organic hemp throw rugs in a variety of colors)
- **Ten Thousand Villages:** www.tenthousandvillages.com (handmade, fair trade–certified rugs and floor mats)

Also, consider buying an Oriental rug. Typically they are made from natural fibers, such as wool, silk, cotton, goat's hair, and camel's hair, with wool being the most popular material for the pile of the rug.

A product called AFM SafeChoice Carpet Seal is designed to prevent the out-gassing of harmful chemicals used in carpet backing glues and from the padding below. It is odor-free and effectively blocks out-gassing for up to five cleanings or 1 year. It is designed to be used in conjunction with SafeChoice Carpet Shampoo (to clean) and SafeChoice Lock Out (to seal carpet fibers and repel dirt and stains). These products are not recommended for wool carpets; they are available at several online sites, including www.greenest.com.

FLOORS

Floors cover a lot of surface area in your home, so it's important to consider the materials they are made of. Whether you have old wooden floors or new, there are things to consider. A study published in 2008 revealed that old wood floor finishes in some homes may be a source of exposure to the now-banned environmental pollutants polychlorinated biphenyls (PCBs). PCBs are persistent organic pollutants that have been found in human blood and breast milk. They affect the immune, reproductive, nervous, and endocrine systems and are associated with thyroid toxicity as well as breast cancer. Research by the Silent Spring Institute showed that current exposure from old wood floor finishes may be an even more significant source of PCBs for some people than diet. When finishing your wood floors, look for a nontoxic product such as Tried & True Wood Finishes (eg, linseed oil–based Original Wood Finish, $16/quart).

If you choose to install new wood floors, make sure that the wood carries the seal of approval from the Forest Stewardship Council (FSC). They certify that wood products such as flooring (and furniture) have been harvested by using certified sustainable standards.

If you'd like an alternative to wood, consider bamboo or cork, both of which are priced comparably to hardwoods. Bamboo is durable, resistant to insects and moisture, and eco-friendly because the bamboo plant reaches maturity in a lot less time than the trees harvested to make wood floors. Make sure you find a manufacturer that doesn't use lamination glues that contain formaldehyde.

3 WAYS TO MAKE A SHIFT

1. Try recycled modular carpeting. This helps avert some of the 1.8 million tons of rugs and carpeting sent to landfills each year. It is about three times as expensive as regular carpet, but you can keep it longer by replacing sections. Flor is one company that offers recycled modular carpeting.

2. Consider natural linoleum. Marmoleum looks like old-fashioned linoleum, but it's made by using linseed oil, tree rosin, lime, and other natural materials.

Remove your Shoes

In most Asian homes, removing the shoes at the front door is a common tradition and a symbol of respect. Here in America, it's not so common, but it's something I've been trying to create as a habit in my own home. Shoes track in lead, pesticides, and other pollutants that contaminate our carpets and floors. Stuff we track in from the outside can turn our homes into toxic places, especially for pets and young children, who spend more time on the floor.

If you don't take off your shoes, consider wiping them on a door mat. Or set aside an entryway closet specifically for storing your shoes when you enter the house. If you enter from the garage, a shoe rack at the door makes it easy. You can always offer slippers to those who want to put something on their feet. Here are some benefits of removing your shoes:

- Leaving your shoes at the door can be a symbol of leaving behind the harried world outside.

- Less dirt and fewer pollutants are brought in from the outside.

- Going barefoot feels good and is good for your circulation.

- You'll spend less time cleaning the floor.

- Infants, young children, and pets will inhale cleaner indoor air.

Save the Cork!

The sound of a cork popping out of a bottle is often synonymous with joy and celebration. But do you know where cork actually comes from and what it really is? Cork is the bark of the cork oak tree, which renews itself after harvesting; not a single tree is cut down. These trees are a vital source of income for thousands of people in countries such as Portugal, Spain, Italy, and France.

The WWF (World Wildlife Fund) released a report saying that up to 75 percent of the cork forests in the Mediterranean might be lost within the next 10 years—all because of plastic screw-top wine bottles. By the year 2015, only 5 percent of wine bottles may be using cork. Without protection of the cork forests, habitat and livelihoods may be lost.

Recycling programs are just starting up around the country to recycle the cork stoppers and turn them into cork flooring. Another way to use your old wine corks is to buy a wine cork trivet kit. You take eight wine corks and screw them onto coils that come in the kit, making a ready-to-use recycled hot plate. The kit is available at www.replayground.com.

3. Check out bamboo or cork flooring. Teragren is a brand of durable bamboo flooring, and Habitus is a cork flooring made from wine stopper waste.

WALLS

A few years ago, I wallpapered a room in my home and was bombarded by a noxious odor, kind of like the smell of a new beach ball. Then I noticed a similar odor when I hung a new plastic shower curtain liner. I did some digging and found out that the bad smell comes from volatile organic compounds (VOCs), those airborne chemicals or gases (formaldehyde, xylene, and toluene) that I spoke about earlier. As you may recall, those with weakened immune systems, chemical sensitivities, or asthma, as well as young children and the elderly, are particularly susceptible to the effects of breathing in VOCs.

In 2008, researchers at the Virginia-based Center for Health, Environment & Justice released findings from their study on what caused the new shower curtain smell. They tested the chemical composition of unopened PVC (polyvinyl chloride) plastic shower curtains bought from Bed Bath & Beyond, Kmart, Sears, Target, and Walmart. The study found that the curtains contained high concentrations of phthalates; one of the curtains released measurable quantities of as many as 108 VOCs into the air, some of which persisted for nearly a month. Very little information on toxicity is available for 86 of the 108 chemicals detected in the curtains.

According to the Center for Health, Environment & Justice, VOCs are always emitted from those easy-to-clean wallpapers made from PVC, referred to simply as "vinyl." And since wall coverings cover a lot more surface area than you think, they can have a big negative effect on your indoor air quality. Unknowingly, we buy what we think looks good rather than what's safe.

The general consensus in the healthy-building world is that PVC is reasonably suspected of being linked to disruption of the endocrine system, reproductive impairment, impaired child development and birth defects, neurotoxicity, immune system suppression, and even cancer. "With PVC, we are most concerned with soft, flexible products that cover large surface areas and are in direct contact with the airstream of a home. That's wallpaper and vinyl flooring," explains John Dunnihoo, general manager of Healthy Home Plans in northern California. "We don't lose too much sleep at night worrying about the vinyl insulation wrap on electrical wiring that is hidden in the wall cavity. However, we are concerned with any plastic products, including PVC, [that are] outside and exposed to the sun, like vinyl siding, [and] vinyl gutters."

There are natural alternatives to vinyl. The environmental organization Greenpeace recommends paper-based wallpaper, with recycled and biodegradable being the best choices. Other natural fibers to look for include linen, cotton, silk, sisal (extracted from leaves of the agave plant), cork, rice paper, grasscloth, jute (finely split bamboo), and cellulose (wood pulp). Check the materials list before you buy because some manufacturers blend natural fibers with vinyl or PVC. Natural wall coverings are not cheap: They can cost between $35 and $60 a yard.

Installation using traditional wallpaper paste is preferable to using self-stick wall coverings because of the high levels of VOC content in the adhesive. In general, the smoother the surface is, the cleaner it stays and the easier it is to clean. Paper coated with liquid acrylic (make sure you don't get liquid vinyl) is wipeable; uncoated paper wallpaper wouldn't be practical for a kitchen, nursery, or child's room, for example.

Wall covering with a woven or rough texture requires more adhesive to hold it to the wall, so a no-VOC adhesive becomes doubly important. If you haven't wallpapered before or your walls are uneven (as they are in many older houses), you may want to consider professional installation. Either way, allow a few days for the room to air out afterward.

WHAT YOU SHOULD KNOW

- According to the EPA, PVC is a known human carcinogen. It's so toxic, in fact, that it is banned in some parts of Europe.

- Greenpeace says, "PVC is the most dangerous of all plastics, and its manufacture is linked to the production of chlorine to a degree unmatched by any other material."

- If you've got vinyl wallpaper in high-moisture areas in your home, it can create a vapor barrier that traps moisture in the wall and encourages mold growth. It can also harbor mildew in hot, humid climates when air conditioning is used.

If you'd like to learn more about the dangers of vinyl, check out the documentary "Blue Vinyl" at www.bluevinyl.org. It's an eye-opening investigative journey about the vinyl siding used on millions of homes in America. The filmmaker shows how truly toxic it is to PVC factory workers as well as to our environment.

3 WAYS TO MAKE A SHIFT

1. Choose paper-based wallpaper instead of vinyl. Other natural fibers to consider include linen, cotton, sisal, cork, grasscloth, and cellulose.

2. Use traditional wallpaper paste instead of self-stick wall coverings. Self-stick adhesives contain high levels of VOCs.

3. After installing wall covering, allow a few days for the room to air out. Think about hiring a professional to do the job, especially if you haven't wallpapered before or your walls are uneven.

Where to Shop

Dozens of companies make environmentally friendly wall coverings using natural, nontoxic ingredients. Look for them at local green furniture stores as well as online:

- **DesignTex has EarthTex,** a non-PVC wall covering without heavy metals or plasticizers: www.dtex.com
- **Hollingsworth & Vose has WallTek,** a line of nonwoven wall coverings containing no PVC or formaldehyde: www.hollingsworth-vose.com
- **Innovations in Wallcoverings, Inc.,** has a line of natural, renewable, recyclable, and biodegradable materials; they use water-based inks containing no heavy metals: www.innovationsusa.com
- **MDC Wallcoverings** offers Natural Environments, which use natural materials, including the dyes: www.mdcwall.com
- **Natural Cork** sells cork wall tiles, which are often used like wallpaper: www.naturalcork.com
- **Newcastle Fabrics** has the South Seas collection, which is natural: www.newcastlefabrics.com
- **Roos International** offers Texturglas products, which use a specially formulated adhesive called Ecofix (a starch-based powder made from regenerated, degradable materials, creating no VOC emissions): www.roosintl.com
- **Sinan Company Environmental Products** makes a plant-based wallpaper adhesive called 389 Natural Wallpaper Adhesive: www.sinanco.com
- **Wolf-Gordon, Inc.,** has an Ecological Reclamation Program with its EarthSafe collection called Strata, made of natural, renewable, or recyclable materials and cellulose harvested from managed forests; at the end of the product's life cycle, the wall coverings can be returned (for credit): www.wolf-gordon.com

PAINT

When it comes to paint, look for "low-VOC" or "no-VOC" on the label. There are several decent brands of eco-paints on the market, but they cost a lot more than conventional paints—at least $30 to $35 per gallon. Make sure that the paint you buy carries the Green Seal "mark of environmental responsibility" or meets Green Seal Standard GS-11. The Green Seal organization sets more stringent standards than the EPA for acceptable VOC levels in paint. For example, for interior flat paint, the EPA allows 250 grams per liter (g/L), while Green Seal allows only 50 g/L. The lower VOC level means the paint will have minimal impact on the environment throughout its life cycle, from manufacturing to disposal.

Toxic Black Mold Can Come from Water Damage in Your Home

A friend of mine recently returned from a trip to England where she visited her in-laws' home. The bedroom she slept in shared a wall with an indoor swimming pool. The noise of its generator forced my friend to use ear plugs, which she'd remove in the morning and place on a night table next to the bed. Within 2 days she developed pain in her ear that forced her to go to the emergency department.

The doctors told her she had *Aspergillus niger*, a toxic black mold that invaded her ear canal. It also traveled into one of her lungs, showing up as a spot on a scan. She was told she probably contracted the condition from the home she was visiting. When they peeled away the wallpaper from the wall next to her bed, it revealed black mold.

Inhaling or touching this mold can be dangerous to your health. As molds multiply, they release mycotoxins into the air—toxins produced by the fungus that can act as irritants or allergens and wreak havoc on your health, especially if you're sensitive. Some types of mycotoxins can cause disease or serious health problems. The night table in the bedroom had been covered with these invisible mycotoxins, which attached themselves to my friend's ear plugs. She now has permanent hearing loss in one of her ears, as well as tinnitus, or constant ringing in her ears.

According to the *Journal of the American Medical Association* (JAMA), mold growth in water-damaged homes is a potential hazard and can be a serious health risk. Dampness in basements, walls, carpets, and wood caused by flooding provides an excellent environment for molds to flourish. If you've had a flood or excessive moisture in your home, check for evidence of mold—the organisms multiply very fast.

When we moved into our home a few years ago, we had a flood in one of our bathrooms. Because I knew the possibility that toxic mold could develop quickly, we hired an environmental team to inspect the damage. Within 48 hours we had black mold growing on our dry wall, which meant that parts of the walls needed to be replaced.

One example of paint meeting the Green Seal standard is Freshaire from Home Depot; another is Harmony by Sherwin-Williams. To get an even lower VOC content you'll need to find either nontoxic or natural paint, which tends to be even more expensive. Smaller manufacturers such as Yolo Colorhouse, available at Home Depot, and Mythic Paint, available at certain independent paint stores, sell only low- or no-VOC paints. In addition to their own colors, they say they can match any color from a large paint manufacturer, like Benjamin Moore.

There is a new alternative paint product available called ceramic paint that provides both low VOC and high durability. Ceramic Coat by O'Leary Paint comes with antimicrobial protection. This paint is touted as healthy, able to withstand scrubbing without losing its flat finish, and able to prevent mold, mildew, and bacteria from growing.

In 2008, *Consumer Reports* magazine assessed 57 interior paints currently on the market, including low-VOC ones. Paints were rated on their ability to hide imperfections, surface smoothness, ease of cleaning, and gloss change and fading. The low-VOC paints were given "mixed marks." At the top was Benjamin Moore's Aura, which ranked third among 21 paints in the low-luster category; True Value EasyCare and Glidden Evermore came in sixth and seventh, respectively.

Earth911.com is a great Web site where you can find out where to recycle or donate leftover paint. Also check out their paint calculators, which can help you buy just the amount you need.

Natural Paint Manufacturers

- **AFM (American Formulating & Manufacturing):** www.afmsafecoat.com (SafeCoat, low-VOC and no-VOC paints and primer sealers)
- **American Clay:** www.americanclay.com (made from natural clays and vibrant natural pigments)
- **American Pride Paints:** www.americanpridepaint.com (great for people with chemical sensitivities)
- **Anna Sova:** www.annasova.com (made from 99% food-grade ingredients)
- **BioShield:** www.bioshieldpaint.com (both matte and gloss finishes, plus all-natural primer and thinner)
- **C2 LoVo non-toxic line:** www.c2paint.com
- **California Paints Elements Zero VOC:** www.californiapaints.com (uses Mircoban technology for keeping paint free of mold and stains)
- **Freshaire Choice Paint:** www.freshairechoice.com (no-VOC paint)

- **Mythic nontoxic, low-odor paint:** www.mythicpaint.com
- **Old-Fashioned Real Milk Paint Company:** www.milkpaint.com (milk-based paints with natural pigments)
- **Serena and Lily:** www.serenaandlily.com/paint (designed especially for kids' and babies' rooms; low VOC, low odor, and mold resistant)
- **Yolo Colorhouse:** www.yolocolorhouse.com (low- or no-VOC paint)

Green Seal–Certified Paint Manufacturers

- **Benjamin Moore,** Pristine Eco-Spec Interior line
- **Cloverdale Paint,** Horizon Interior line
- **Devoe,** Wonder-Pure No-VOC/Odor
- **Duron,** Genesis Odor-Free
- **Dutch Boy,** Clarity Interior Latex line
- **Glidden/ICI,** ProMaster Low-Odor
- **HealthyHome.com,** HealthyHues Interior Latex line
- **Kelly-Moore,** Enviro-Cote
- **MAB Paints,** Enviro-Pure Interior Latex Zero VOC line
- Miller Paint Co., Acro Solvent Free Interior Acrylic line
- **Olympic Paint and Stain,** Zero-VOC Olympic Premium Interior line—low-odor and widely available at Lowe's
- **Pittsburgh Paints/PPG,** Pure Performance and Speedhide Low Odor
- **Rodda Paint Company,** Horizon Interior line
- **Sherwin-Williams,** Harmony/HealthSpec Low Odor
- **Sico Inc.,** Ecosource and Expert lines
- **Southern Diversified Products,** American Pride and American Pro lines
- **Vista Paint,** Carefree Earth Coat line

UPHOLSTERED FURNITURE

Take a look at the materials in the furniture you've chosen for your home. That comfy upholstered couch you're sitting on is probably coated in polybrominated diphenylethers, or PBDEs, flame-retardant chemicals designed to slow a

Green Office Furniture Options

- Knoll has been awarded LEED certification for its furniture. www.knoll.com

- Ecowork offers eco-friendly furniture using sustainable materials and processes. It is a member of the US Green Building Council. www.ecowork.com

- Steelcase is the first office furniture manufacturer to initiate large-scale testing of its office furniture products for indoor air quality impact. www.steelcase.com

- Guilford of Maine boasts that 98 percent of its fabrics are made entirely of recycled polyester or bio-based yarns. guilfordofmaine.com

fire and provide adequate time for escape. When the environmental group Friends of the Earth tested samples from 350 pieces of household furniture, they found that most had high levels of these fire retardants.

PBDEs are life-saving chemicals, but they may actually be making you sick. They are linked to cancer, birth defects, learning disabilities, and other health issues in humans and in pets. Animal studies have shown that high levels of exposure interfere with thyroid hormone, which is essential for healthy brain development. There is now an epidemic of thyroid disease among house cats in the United States, and scientists reported in 2007 that it may be linked to exposure to flame retardants. Perhaps cats are our live-in sentinels!

Several states have banned the use of certain flame retardants based on biomonitoring studies conducted by Mount Sinai School of Medicine in New York City, in collaboration with the Environmental Working Group. Other states are preparing to follow suit.

WHAT YOU SHOULD KNOW

- When buying furniture, you can't tell from the label whether it contains flame retardants. They are sprayed on the foam cushions inside all kinds of upholstery. You need to ask the sales person.

- The chemicals in flame retardants don't stay put in your furniture. They go into the air and the dust in your home.

- PBDEs have been found in human breast milk and dryer lint.

3 WAYS TO MAKE A SHIFT

1. Before buying new upholstered furniture, ask the sales staff whether your prospective sofa or chair contains "halogenated fire retardants." If it's made from polyurethane foam, it most likely contains fire retardants that can easily leach. Look for a style in which the foam is thickly covered or wrapped inside the cushion, so dust is less likely to escape into your home.

2. Ask if the manufacturer offers nontoxic stain-resistant fabrics, or look for Nano-Tex, a new technology that doesn't coat the fabric.

3. Look for the Greenguard and the Green Seal (www.greenguard.org, or www.greenseal.org) logos.

WOOD FURNITURE

If your tables, chairs, desk, and cabinets are made of plywood or particle board, chances are they have been treated with pesticides and constructed with glue that contains formaldehyde. As I mentioned earlier, formaldehyde is a carcinogen, and inhaling its vapors can cause headaches, insomnia, and respiratory problems. Formaldehyde products usually emit vapors for 7 to 8 years, with the greatest intensity during the first year.

New preliminary research suggests that exposure to formaldehyde could greatly increase a person's chances of developing Lou Gehrig's disease, or amyotrophic lateral sclerosis, a progressive, usually fatal disease caused by the degeneration of the nerve cells in the central nervous system that control voluntary muscle movement. "It is estimated that 10 to 20 percent of the US population, including asthmatics, may have hyper-reactive airways, which may make them more susceptible to formaldehyde's effects," reports the EPA booklet "Indoor Air Pollution."

Japan, Europe, and China restrict formaldehyde in wood furniture products because of health concerns. "But the US has no federal limits on formaldehyde in consumer products, so cabinets in schools and homes across the nation can contain unlimited amounts of the cancer-causing

Do-it-yourself formaldehyde test kits are available by mail. Or you can hire an environmental testing firm to check whether the chemical is present in your home (www.indoorairtest.com or www.sylvane.com).

chemical," says Stacy Malkan, author of *Not Just a Pretty Face: The Ugly Side of the Beauty Industry.*

Also, if your wood furniture was manufactured within the past 20 years, it probably came from a forest that is endangered. More than 80 percent of the world's old growth (ancient trees) has already been cut down, with much of it ending up in everyday furniture. Experts say that these forests, filled with wildlife and herbal remedies, will vanish within the next 10 to 15 years if our current logging practice continues. You can help prevent this from happening by choosing alternatives and following the advice below.

3 WAYS TO MAKE A SHIFT

1.. Look for the FSC seal of approval from the Forest Stewardship Council or find a manufacturer that uses salvaged and reclaimed wood from urban trees and old buildings.

2. Try furniture made from bamboo, which is strong and harvested from sustainable sources. Another option is biocomposite boards, which are made from wheat, sorghum, rice, and sunflower.

3. Air out new furniture in a well-ventilated space, or buy used furniture or antiques, which may no longer be emitting VOCs.

Friends of the Earth suggests taking additional steps to make the healthiest, most environmentally friendly choices when furnishing your home:

- Buy wooden furniture or furniture filled with polyester, down, wool, or cotton. It is unlikely to contain added fire-retardant chemicals.

- Vacuum often and use a HEPA filter to keep the dust level down in your house.
- Look for all-wool linings and latex filling, both of which are fire-safe and free of fire-retardant chemicals.

Where to Shop

Products with the FSC logo are available from a variety of manufacturers, including home improvement stores such as Home Depot and Lowe's. Crate and Barrel sells some eco-friendly sofas and chairs at fairly reasonable prices. There are also lots of eco-friendly online furniture sites. Some of my favorites are:

- **InMod:** www.inmod.com
- **Maria Yee:** www.inhabitat.com
- **Vivavi:** www.vivavi.com

Also, Ethan Allen is launching an eco-friendly furniture line in early 2009.

Furniture Companies That Use FSC-Certified or Reclaimed Wood

- **Berkeley Mills:** www.berkeleymills.com
- **Cisco Brothers Furniture,** Basal Living Collection line: www.ciscobrothers.com
- **Green Sage Furniture:** www.greensage.com
- **The Joinery:** www.thejoinery.com
- **Montauk Furniture:** www.montauksofa.com
- **Urban Hardwoods:** www.urbanhardwoods.com
- **Verellen Home Collection:** www.verellenhc.com
- **Woodshanti:** www.woodshanti.com

AIR PURIFIERS/AIR FILTERS

Buying the right purifier for your home can be confusing. Let me simplify things for you. There are four main types of console-type air purifiers on the market right now; many use a combination of purifying techniques.

1. HEPA air purifiers: These use pleated high-efficiency air particulate (HEPA) filters, developed by the U.S. Atomic Energy Commission to screen out and trap sub-micron particles. Many reviews say this type of air purifier is the most effective.

2. Electronic ionizers or ion generators: These use a process to electrically charge airborne particles, which are then attracted to collection plates in the air purifier. The particles can also be deposited on your clothing and furniture.

3. UV purifiers: These rely on ultraviolet (UV) light to neutralize biological contaminants. UV light is effective in destroying microbes such as bacteria, dust mites, and mold spores, given sufficient exposure time.

4. Ozone generators: These do not remove allergens from the air. Instead, they release ozone, which in large amounts can neutralize strong odors (such as the smoke odor from fire damage).

According to the EPA, ozone is considered a toxic gas and can cause lung damage and exacerbate asthma symptoms. It also can react with household cleaners on your kitchen countertop, or air fresheners you've sprayed, and then produce harmful secondary chemicals such as formaldehyde. The U.S. Consumer Product Safety Commission hasn't set ozone limits for such home air purifiers, but the FDA set a limit of 50 parts per billion for medical devices. The California Air Resources Board said that home units generally produce

Consciousness in Candles

Most candles, unless otherwise labeled, are made from paraffin, a petroleum product, that the American Lung Association says emits 11 documented toxins. Fumes from paraffin wax have caused kidney and bladder tumors in laboratory animals. Instead of paraffin candles, choose beeswax candles with cotton wicks (make sure they don't have a lead core, which will release into the air). There are two types of beeswax candles: solid, which are dipped or molded and burn well; and rolled, made from sheets of beeswax and tend to burn more quickly. Another good choice is soy candles. Avoid scented candles because artificial scents emit toxic chemicals as by-products when they burn. For fragrance, essential oils are your best bet. Check the Recommended Resources for places to buy them online.

Blocking/Absorbing Offensive Chemicals

If you are unable to remove furniture, carpeting, or other home furnishings that off-gas, these three strategies can help clear the air:

1. Use an air purifier or air filtration device.

2. Try carbon blankets.

3. Add lots of houseplants to your indoor space.

levels way above that—250 to 500 parts per billion. California recently became the first state to pass a law regulating ozone emissions from all types of residential air purifiers. Starting in 2010, no machine intended for home use may produce an ozone concentration higher than 50 ppb.

Reviews from *Consumer Reports* magazine and Air Purifiers America say to look for the following in an air cleaner:

- A clean air delivery rate (CADR) that matches the size of the room to be cleaned. Not all manufacturers have submitted their models for CADR testing.

- A HEPA filter with the word "true" in front of the name. Otherwise it could be a lower-grade filter that doesn't trap as many pollutants.

- Air purifiers with fans, which work better in tests.

- A filter monitor that alerts you when the filter needs to be changed. Proper maintenance is crucial for effectiveness.

- Models with different fan speeds, so you can control the noise level. *Consumer Reports* suggests buying a larger unit than you need for a bedroom, then running it on low speed to cut down on noise.

If you choose an electrostatic ionizer, you need to dust or vacuum regularly to actually remove the allergens from your living space. Also, be aware that most electrostatic devices produce a small amount of toxic ozone as a byproduct.

Personally, I don't have an air filter in my home; I live in a mild climate, so I can keep my windows open. But I do use a vacuum with a HEPA filter, and I change the pleated air return filters in my furnace every 3 months.

You can find air purifiers online at:

Houseplants

NASA has been studying the effects of plants on air quality for about 20 years; their research confirms that common houseplants are natural air purifiers. While the original research was aimed at finding ways to purify the air for extended stays in orbiting space stations, the findings are important for us on Earth as well. The following plants are documented as being especially good at improving indoor air quality:

- Aloe vera: formaldehyde
- Areca palm: all indoor air toxins
- Elephant ear philodendron: formaldehyde
- Lady palm: all indoor air toxins
- Bamboo or reed palm: benzene, trichloroethylene, and formaldehyde
- Rubber plant: formaldehyde
- Dracaena 'Janet Craig' (corn plant): benzene and cigarette smoke
- English ivy: benzene and formaldehyde
- Dwarf date palm: xylene (found in paints, solvents and adhesives)
- Ficus (weeping fig): formaldehyde
- Boston fern: formaldehyde
- Peace lily: acetone, trichloroethylene, benzene, and formaldehyde
- Golden pothos: carbon monoxide, benzene, and formaldehyde
- Kimberley Queen fern: formaldehyde
- Florist's mums (chrysanthemum): formaldehyde, benzene, and ammonia
- Gerbera daisy: all indoor toxins
- Dragon tree (*Dracaena marginata*): xylene and trichloroethylene
- Red emerald philodendron: all indoor air toxins
- Parlor palm: all indoor air toxins
- Spider plant: carbon monoxide

- **AirFree Air Purifiers:** www.airfree.com
- **Air Purifiers America:** www.air-purifiers-america.com
- **AllerAir:** www.allerair.com
- **ClearFlite:** www.airpurifiers.com
- **Gaiam:** www.gaiam.com (see their germ-free humidifier, too)
- **Ultra-Pure:** www.ultra-pureair.com

Carbon Blankets and Sealants

There is a product on the market that will absorb the chemicals and fumes from things such as sofas and carpets. It's called a carbon blanket or carbon felt fabric, and as its name suggests, it contains activated carbon, which has been processed to make it extremely porous. These blankets can be used in new cars and, when traveling, for covering hotel mattresses. The blankets and fabric are reusable and can be reactivated—the blankets by placing them in the hot sun for a few hours, and the fabric in a hot dryer. They can be purchased at Nirvana Safe Haven in Walnut Creek, California, or online at the store's Web site: www.nontoxic.com.

AFM Hardseal and Safeseal (maker of Safecoat natural paint) are liquids that dry clear and seal in odors and chemical off-gassing. They can be used on furniture and wood flooring. Hardseal has a gloss finish and can be used both on porous and nonporous surfaces. Safeseal is for porous surfaces; it dries to a matte finish that is almost invisible.

CLEARING THE AIR OF CELL PHONE RADIATION

There's no doubt we live in a digital age. Studies from around the world are now being released with some startling news about using cell phones. A 2007 Swedish study reports that radio waves from mobile phones penetrate deep into the brain, not just around the ear. Researchers found that using a cell phone for 10 years or longer will double the risk of getting an acoustic neuroma, a tumor on a nerve that connects the ear to the brain. Children, because they have thinner skulls than adults and nervous systems that are still developing, are particularly vulnerable.

A 2008 study involving more than 13,000 children, conducted at UCLA and Aarhus University in Denmark, took even the scientists behind it by surprise. They found that mothers who used cell phones while they were pregnant

Portable Air Purity

The AirPod personal air purifier by Blueair is a compact system that looks like an iPod, weighs less than 2 pounds, cleans the air in a 5' × 6' room, and does not produce ozone. Available from Blueair Store: www.blueairstore.com.

Polluted Pets

Our dogs and cats are not immune from the chemicals in our homes. They spend most of their days in direct contact with our floors and carpets, while some of the lucky ones are sleeping on our couches and chairs.

In April 2008, the Environmental Working Group released data showing concentrations of chemicals in pets that were more than 20 times what's been detected in the typical adult human. They found 35 chemicals in the dogs and 46 in the cats they studied. Cats had 23 times the amount of brominated flame retardants (used in furniture, fabrics, and electronics) in humans, while dogs had 2.4 times the levels of perfluorinated chemicals (from stain- and grease-proof coatings).

Like cats and dogs, small children spend lots of time on the ground, so for the sake of all your little critters, make healthy choices in your home.

Check out eco-friendly, nontoxic pet toys and beds at:

- **EcoAnimal:** www.ecoanimal.com
- **Pristine Planet:** www. pristineplanet.com
- **West Paw Design:** www. westpawdesign.com

were 54 percent more likely to have children with behavioral problems when they reached school age. When the children later used cell phones themselves, they were, overall, 80 percent more likely to suffer from difficulties with behavior. Specifically, they were 25 percent more at risk from emotional problems, 34 percent more likely to suffer from difficulties relating to their peers, 35 percent more likely to be hyperactive, and 49 percent more prone to problems with conduct.

Short-term cell phone use can also have adverse effects. Scientists at the Spanish Neuro Diagnostic Research Institute in Marbella conducted a 10-year study, released in May 2008, which showed that a call lasting just 2 minutes can alter the natural electrical activity of a child's brain for up to an hour afterwards. Doctors fear that disturbed brain activity in children could affect their mood and ability to learn and lead to psychiatric and behavioral problems. Another study released in 2008, conducted at the Massachusetts Institute of Technology (MIT), showed that college and MBA students who were exposed to cell phone electromagnetic radiation had disturbed sleep patterns, potentially affecting the body's ability to recover from stress.

Britain's advisory body on radiologic hazards, the Health Protection Agency, has urged parents to limit their children's use of cell phones, recommending that younger children use cell phones only in emergencies. Here in the United States, there are no precautionary guidelines, and toy companies are teaming up with wireless companies and marketing to kids as young as five. For example, LeapFrog's "TicTalk" and Mattel's "My Scene" are simple phones with five speed-dial buttons—kind of a cross between a phone and a pager. As kids get older and are exposed to more advanced phones, they'll surely be pressuring parents for an upgrade. Also, I'm aware that kids aren't just using their phones to talk. They're text messaging, taking pictures, playing video games, and surfing the Web, which opens up a whole new set of concerns.

Cell phones have certainly become a big part of life. There are over three billion of them in use on our planet. According to a 2005 survey by the ad agency BBDO Worldwide, 75 percent of American cell phone owners had it turned on and within reach during their waking hours, 59 percent wouldn't think of lending their cell phone to a friend for a day, and 26 percent said it was more important to go home to retrieve a cell phone than a wallet. About half of American teens ages 13 to 16 have a cell phone, and now companies have set their sights on 9- to 12-year-olds, or "tweens," as the next untapped market for cell phone use. But before you're persuaded to go out and buy your child a cell phone, think twice before hooking them up.

Bottom line? Do what brain surgeons do: In 2008 three prominent neurosurgeons told CNN's Larry King that they did not hold cell phones next to their ears. Keith Black, MD, a surgeon at Cedars-Sinai Medical Center in Los Angeles, Vini Khurana, PhD, an associate professor of neurosurgery at the Australian National University, and CNN's chief medical correspondent, Dr. Sanjay Gupta, a neurosurgeon at Emory University Hospital, said they use ear pieces instead.

Cell Phones and the Environment

According to the EPA, Americans discard 125 million phones each year, creating 65,000 tons of waste. These old phones—many containing hazardous materials such as lead, mercury, cadmium, flame retardants, and arsenic—are now the fastest-growing type of manufactured garbage in the nation.

3 WAYS TO MAKE A SHIFT

1. Use a hollow tube headset* or speaker phone whenever you or your child uses a cell phone.

2. Before making a call, check the number of bars that indicate reception. A good signal means that the phone is using less radiation to transmit.

3. Consider attaching a chip or shield to your phone to reduce the effects of EMR (electromagnetic radiation). Several companies offer these; they can be found online at www.sarshield.com, www.cellphonedefense.com, and www.waveshield.com, as well as at Target.

Where There's Smoke . . .

You may be surprised to learn (I know I was!) that those wrapped, factory-produced fake logs are actually healthier to burn than real wooden logs. The problem with wood isn't the wood, it's the smoke. Smoke is made up of fine particles called particulate matter, which is unhealthy to breathe. It can cause burning eyes and even bronchitis and can aggravate chronic heart and lung diseases.

Also, when wood smoke is released through the chimney, it becomes air pollution. In 2006, the EPA released a study comparing emissions from real logs and fake ones. It showed that the carbon monoxide emission rate of artificial logs is around 75 percent less than that of real wood, and that artificial logs create 80 percent less particulate matter. Artificial logs will also warm your home more efficiently.

Duraflame, the largest manufacturer of fire logs, has now gone green. They switched from using petroleum-based waxes as a binder to vegetable paraffin. It's also pretty cost-effective: a 6-pound Duraflame log lasts about 3½ hours, which the company says is the equivalent of burning 30 pounds of firewood.

One of the coolest fake logs on the market is called the Java Log, made from old coffee grounds. The manufacturer gets the old grounds from companies that make instant coffee, diverting 20 million pounds of coffee waste from landfills. Natural vegetable wax is used to hold the grounds together. Coffee has a higher heat density than wood, so these actually burn hotter than wood logs. Available from Java Products: www.java-log.com.

---

* A hollow tube headset uses a flexible plastic tube instead of a wire to transmit the sound from a small speaker to the earpiece. My research suggests that this is the safest type of headset.

UNSUNG HERO

Rafael Pelli is the architect who designed the first green high-rise apartment building in America. Starting about 10 years ago, Rafael had the vision to create a building using only the safest, most natural materials like Forest Stewardship Council (FSC)–certified wood flooring, bamboo kitchen cabinets, carpets without toxic backing or adhesives, and eco-friendly paint.

The Solaire was the first of his three state-of-the-art towers in downtown Manhattan's Battery Park City. Working with the Albanese Organization developer, all of the buildings were constructed using low or no off-gassing materials. They also contain the first onsite water recycling system built in an urban multi-family structure.

Each unit has filtered water from all faucets, showers, and tubs, and filtered air that is automatically cooled and dehumidified in summer, heated and humidified in winter. In addition, there is solar paneling as well as pesticide-free rooftop gardens.

Growing up in the 1960s in Los Angeles had a big influence on Rafael. He appreciated the beauty of the land but was also affected by LA's poor air quality. "As a kid I got pain in my chest running around in the smog," he said. "When I moved to New York I realized smog isn't normal! It made me keenly aware of my environment." When he became an architect, he felt passionate about creating buildings that didn't negatively affect the environment, were energy efficient, and contributed to people's health and well-being.

In 1990, Rafael joined his father's architectural firm Pelli Clarke Pelli and now runs their New York office. For more information: www.thesolaire.com.

Chapter 9

THE KITCHEN, LAUNDRY ROOM, AND BATHROOM

Discover Safe Household Cleaners, Cookware, and Dishware

"I hate housework. You make the beds, you wash the dishes and six months later you have to start all over again."

—JOAN RIVERS

SALLY IS A WELL-MEANING WOMAN who, in trying to protect her family from germs, takes clean to extreme. When I visited her home one day, I noticed that she was using copious amounts of disinfectant wipes and sprays, scented antibacterial soap, and fragranced laundry detergent. She also burns lots of scented candles. Sally thinks her house smells "clean and fresh"; to me it smells like a chemical plant.

In her quest to keep her home spotless and her family healthy, Sally wipes and sprays her kitchen and bathroom surfaces, her children's toys, and even their fingers, with things she considers to be safe, effective cleaning products. In actuality, she might unsuspectingly be causing health problems right in her own home. One of her sons has severe allergies, and the other has asthma. Is it possible that their medical problems could be caused or exacerbated by her cleaning products? There are those who think so.

Researchers around the world are finding links between the rise in the "cleanliness factor" and the increase in asthma and allergies. In Great Britain, for example, researchers have found a clear association between childhood asthma and wheezing and the frequent use of common household cleaning products such as bleach, disinfectants, and air fresheners. Children were twice as likely to develop breathing problems if their parents regularly used such products. In 2007, researchers of an international study involving over 3,500 people in 10 European countries said that spraying a cleaner just once a week can trigger an attack, and the risk increases with the frequency of spraying.

It's a bit ironic to think that our cleanliness—the way we over-practice hygiene—actually may contribute to unhealthiness. In many medical circles this is known as the "hygiene hypothesis." First coined by David P. Strachan, MD, in 1989 in an article published in the *British Medical Journal*, the hygiene hypothesis states that too much protection from infectious pathogens weakens a developing immune system. In other words, if your immune system is not challenged early on in life to deal with certain germs, it won't develop properly, and it may become dysfunctional to the point that it's permanently super-sensitive to allergens—many of which would be otherwise harmless.

In recent years, this hypothesis has expanded to include exposure to several varieties of microorganisms and parasites, with which we've coexisted throughout much of our evolutionary history. For millions of years they have been a necessary ingredient in the development of a balanced and healthy immune system. But now modern science and technology may be going too far in removing that critical exposure to these microorganisms and parasites. We could be putting ourselves at risk for downgrading our immune systems, or tripping them out of whack.

Asthma is the leading cause of chronic illness in children, and at the heart of asthma is an immune system that cannot tolerate certain substances. It affects as many as 10 to 12 percent of children in the United States and, for unknown reasons, is steadily increasing. "Asthma has become the leading cause of admission to hospital for children beyond the newborn period," says Philip Landrigan, MD, a New York City pediatrician and co-author of *Raising Children Toxic Free*.

Respiratory conditions such as asthma, pneumonia, and acute bronchitis account for nearly 40 percent of emergency department admissions for infants and toddlers. According to the Centers for Disease Control and Prevention, asthma is the number one reason for school absenteeism in America. It affects more children than any other chronic disease. It's on the rise in adults, too. According to the US Department of Health and Human Services, between 2000 and 2005 the number of adults who were hospitalized and found to have asthma increased from about 753,000 to over 1.6 million—an increase of 113 percent.

There may be something to be said for letting our children play in the mud. Over-protective moms such as Sally might be setting their children up for immune dysfunction. Perhaps asthma or allergies haven't happened in your home yet, or you haven't seen a connection between what you clean with and how it might affect your health, but you can be sure Sally's cleaning scenario is being played out in homes all across the country.

To help prove my point, here's a quote from an online blog in which the writer is addressing the topic of using antibacterial cleaners: "I live on disinfectant wipes and bleach. Bleach has been around for a loooooooooooong time. I doubt it's as dangerous as today's Nazis make it out to be. LOL I would be dead if it were!" Then there's the woman who said: "I also use wipes on a lot of things. No health problems at my house yet!"

Let me ask you this: Why wait for health problems to start? As you become aware of what's inside your cleaning supplies, it will be easier for you to switch to something nontoxic. For example, Lysol Anti-bacterial Action Spray contains alkyl dimethyl benzyl ammonium chloride—a pesticide according to the Environmental Protection Agency (EPA); Clorox Disinfecting Wipes have dimethyl benzyl ammonia chloride and dimethyl ethyl benzyl ammonia chloride—pesticides as well. Do you really want your children and your pets consistently exposed to these heavy-duty chemicals?

On the following pages are suggestions to help you keep your family safe from inhaling indoor air pollutants from your everyday cleaning products.

Ways You Are Exposed to Indoor Air Pollution in Your Home

- Household cleaners
- Dry-cleaning chemicals
- Synthetic fragrances, air fresheners, and aerosol sprays
- Nonstick cookware
- Lead glazes in dishware

HOUSEHOLD CLEANERS

If you've ever walked down the household-cleanser aisle at the supermarket and your eyes began to burn, or your nose became irritated, it's because common cleaning products contain chemicals that can be more dangerous than the germs themselves. Every time your children roll around on the carpet or your pets lick crumbs off the floor, they are being exposed to noxious chemicals.

Don't make the assumption that if it's on the grocery shelf, it has been tested and is safe. Most of us, unwittingly, buy products for our home with ingredients that are either poorly studied or not studied at all, or are known to pose potentially serious health risks. Of the roughly 17,000 chemicals found in common household products, only 3 in 10 have been tested for their effects on human health. Why? Because, just as with cosmetics, the US Consumer Product Safety Commission does not require manufacturers to test household cleaning products before they appear on store shelves.

So if you're reading labels expecting to get the whole picture, know that they provide only limited information. According to the Children's Health Environmental Coalition, a national nonprofit that educates the public on environmental toxins that affect children's health, labels often omit inert ingredients that can make up as much as 90 percent of a product's volume.

Now, the word "inert" doesn't mean inactive or neutral as you might believe. The EPA categorized "inert" ingredients as causing long-term health damage and harm to the environment. These ingredients include solvents, dispersal agents, dyes, and fragrances, some of which can pollute the air and water. Other ingredients that are not mentioned may cause cancer or worsen health problems such as allergies and asthma.

Because of consumer demand for environmentally friendly cleaning products, several large corporations are venturing into the green marketplace. For example, in 2008, Clorox introduced a new line of natural cleaners called

Toxic or Not?

It's often easier to determine that a product is toxic than nontoxic, says consumer advocate Debra Lynn Dadd. "Choosing nontoxic products can be a matter of looking for labels that indicate toxicity, and avoiding those, rather than looking for the word 'nontoxic' on the label," she says.

Green Works. Impressively, Clorox requires that more than 99 percent of its ingredients be natural and based on plants or minerals. In addition, they must be biodegradable, nontoxic to fish, and formulated without animal testing. Companies specializing in green certification are now ranking products on biodegradability, toxicity, sensitization, and other easily measurable parameters, but they haven't established ground rules for what constitutes a natural or naturally derived ingredient.

One good natural product line is called Get Clean, manufactured by Shaklee. This line does not contain hazardous ingredients such as VOCs, benzene, or formaldehyde and is fragrance-free and super-concentrated, which makes the products economical. Shaklee claims their cleaning products out-clean 12 national brands. For more information visit their Web site: www.shaklee.com.

Another terrific all-natural household cleaning line is called Greenwoods Natural, produced by EO Products. See Unsung Heroes below for more information.

WHAT YOU SHOULD KNOW

- The EPA does not require chemical manufacturers to conduct human toxicity studies before approving their chemicals for use in the market. A manufacturer simply has to submit paperwork on a chemical, and wait 90 days for approval.

- While it shouldn't be assumed that because an item is on the shelf it has been tested for safety, you also shouldn't assume that if it says "natural" it's safe. The word "natural" is undefined and unregulated by the government and can be applied to just about anything.

- Since only foods and herbs can be certified organic, the word "organic" on the label of a dish or laundry soap doesn't mean much.

- Most conventional dish and laundry detergents are made from petroleum, a nonrenewable synthetic resource.

3 WAYS TO MAKE A SHIFT

1. Use your nose. If a product smells strong and makes your eyes water, you can bet there's some nasty chemical stuff in the bottle. Remember, cleansers can emit fumes (even while stored) and can affect your home's air quality.

2. Be wary of products that make cleaning too easy. If you don't need to scrub at least a little bit, you should question why.

3. Make your own cleansers. Hydrogen peroxide, vinegar, and baking soda are good alternatives.

Hydrogen Peroxide, Vinegar, and Baking Soda—The Must-Haves

If you're adventurous and you have the time, you can make your own cleaners out of natural, nontoxic ingredients. One thing to have on hand is that plain brown bottle of three-percent hydrogen peroxide sold for less than $1 in any drugstore. It was used medicinally during World War I to help cleanse wounds and kill bacteria in hospitals.

To make your own household cleaner, just fill a spray bottle—preferably made of metal and not plastic—with a 3 percent hydrogen peroxide solution (undiluted) and use it in the kitchen to wipe counter tops and appliances. It will help kill salmonella and other bacteria on wooden cutting boards and will disinfect and give the kitchen a clean, fresh smell. Do the same for the shower to kill bacteria and viruses.

To add even more antigerm power, fill a second bottle with vinegar—either white or apple cider vinegar—and spray one right after the other. It

Easy Alternatives to Harsh Cleansers

Don't use: Bleach.
Use: Borax powder—it can even remove mold. Dilute 1 teaspoon in 1 quart of water and add 2 tablespoons vinegar.

Don't use: Spray furniture polish.
Use: Natural wax polish.

Don't use: Toilet bowl cleaner.
Use: Vinegar. Pour half a 32-ounce bottle into the bowl at night, then scrub away grime in the morning.

Don't use: Oven cleaner.
Use: Natural scrub. Put a heatproof dish filled with water in the oven. Turn on the heat to let the steam soften any baked-on grease. Once the oven is cool, make a paste using equal parts salt, baking soda, and vinegar, and scrub.

Disposing of Household Hazardous Waste

Once you're convinced of the dangers of certain products, you probably will want to throw them away. But it's important to know that you shouldn't throw them into your trash. According to the EPA, "leftover household products that contain corrosive, toxic, ignitable, or reactive ingredients are considered to be 'household hazardous waste.'" Specifically, products such as paints, cleaners, oils, batteries, aerosol products, and pesticides that contain potentially hazardous ingredients require special care when you dispose of them. Call your local sanitation department to see whether they have a hazardous waste disposal program in your neighborhood, or check the EPA's Web site to find one in your area: www.epa.gov/garbage/hhw.htm

doesn't matter which one you use first; you can start with the hydrogen peroxide followed by the vinegar, or the vinegar then the hydrogen peroxide. Just don't mix both liquids in one spray bottle.

In tests performed at Virginia Polytechnic Institute and State University, using the two mists in sequence eliminated almost all *Salmonella*, *E. coli*, and *Shigella* organisms on heavily contaminated foods and surfaces. This spray combination was even more effective at destroying bacteria than any commercially available kitchen cleaner or chlorine bleach.

The disinfectant properties of vinegar have been independently verified by numerous studies, including the Good Housekeeping Institute. A straight five percent solution of vinegar kills 99 percent of bacteria, 82 percent of mold, and 80 percent of viruses.

Don't worry that your home will smell like vinegar; the smell disappears when it dries. Vinegar is also great to clean windows and mirrors. Simply fill a spray bottle with equal parts vinegar and water, then spray away.

Need a substitute for commercial abrasive cleaners? Try baking soda. Put it in a grated-cheese container made of glass with a perforated stainless steel cap (the kind you find at pizza parlors), and just sprinkle it on surfaces and scrub.

Here are more tips for using vinegar and baking soda cleaners:

- To clean nonwood surfaces and tiles, mix 1 cup plain white vinegar with 1 cup water in a spray bottle, and spray the solution onto the surface you want to clean. This mix works as an all-purpose cleaner. Wipe with a moist sponge.

- Use plain, undiluted white vinegar to clean toilets.

- When washing towels, add ½ cup of vinegar to the rinse cycle instead of fabric softener. Fabric softener can make towels less absorbent, but vinegar deodorizes and softens the towels without compromising their absorbency.

- Use baking soda as a scouring powder to clean bathroom sinks, tubs, and showers. For tough stains, form a paste with baking soda and a little bit of water. Smear the paste onto the stain and let it sit for about a half hour, then sponge off.

- Scrub stainless-steel pots and pans with baking soda instead of using scouring pads. Baking soda is nonabrasive, so it doesn't scratch the pans while giving them a nice shine. Baking soda can also be used to clean stainless sinks, and it makes the drain smell better, too! If anything is stuck to the pans or the sink, make a paste of baking soda and water and allow it to sit for 30 minutes before wiping down with a sponge.

- Use baking soda instead of a commercial oven cleaner to clean your oven. When your oven is dirty, apply baking soda and wet it down with water from a spray bottle. Leave it there for 24 hours, occasionally adding more water. Wipe it out with a damp sponge the next day and use a clean, wet cloth to wipe out any remaining residue.

- Use a combination of baking soda and vinegar to loosen up slow drains. Pour ½ cup baking soda into the drain, then slowly and carefully add ½ cup vinegar. Let it sit in the drain for 30 minutes before flushing with hot water.

Source: www.ehow.com

On the Label

Manufacturers are required only to provide hazard symbols such as "poison" and "flammable" and to list main ingredients, not the artificial scents, dyes, and solvents that can make up 90 percent of the volume of a cleaning solution. There are no warnings that say anything like "may cause respiratory problems."

From Soap to Nuts

Did you know there's a laundry soap that grows on trees? They're called soap nuts, and they are made from the dried fruit of the Chinese soapberry tree. A single tree produces hundreds of kilos of nuts per year, which fall to the ground and are collected in Indian and Indonesian forests. The nuts contain saponin, a natural cleaner used for thousands of years to clean clothes in Asia and more recently in Europe. Simply put a few soap nuts into a cotton sack (included in the box it comes in) and drop it in your laundry. Your clothes come out clean, vibrant, and soft. Soap Nuts are 100% biodegradable and are safe for silk and wool. Apparently, they work as a natural fabric softener, too.

LAUNDRY DETERGENTS

Many of the chemicals used in commercially made laundry detergents do not make our clothes clean; they are put there to just make them appear whiter or brighter. Over time, exposure to these chemicals can cause allergies to laundry detergents. In addition, laundry detergents (and fabric softeners) are heavily scented with synthetic chemicals that impart fragrance that remains on our clothing and linens. This residue can be inhaled or can irritate our skin. (I will talk about synthetic fragrances later in this chapter.) The U.S .Consumer Product Safety Commission (CPSC), which regulates household cleaners and determines whether they are toxic, does not consider fragrance ingredients when determining a cleaner's hazard level.

It's best to choose nontoxic laundry detergent that does not contain synthetic perfumes and dyes or chemicals such as chlorine and phosphates that can be irritating to people who have sensitive skin or allergies.

Personally, I like ECOS Earth Friendly brand (Costco sells it), as well as Seventh Generation, BioKleen, and Trader Joe's detergents.

3 WAYS TO MAKE A SHIFT

1. Pick detergents that are biodegradable and contain no phosphates.
2. Instead of bleach, try adding a cup of 3 percent hydrogen peroxide or ½ cup borax for whites, or a cup of white vinegar for darks (it keeps them

from fading). Try a cup of baking soda as a fabric softener. Or use "non-chlorine bleach" cleaning solutions. Fumes from cleansers containing a high concentration of chlorine can irritate the lungs, which is dangerous for those with asthma, emphysema, or a heart condition. The risks are compounded when the cleansers are used in small, poorly ventilated rooms, such as the bathroom. Fragranced chlorine bleaches are even worse because the odor is disguised, which can lead to dangerous overexposure. One product to try instead: Seventh Generation's Non-Chlorine Bleach.

3. Do not use fabric dryer sheets because they contain synthetic chemicals. Instead try lavender sachets from Trader Joe's.

DRY-CLEANING CHEMICALS

Dry-cleaning is called "dry" because water isn't used. Instead, a liquid petroleum-based solvent called perchloroethylene (perc) is the primary cleaning solution. Perc is known to disrupt the central nervous system and contaminate human breast milk.

The U.S. National Institute of Environmental Health Sciences affirms that perc can contribute to headaches, nausea, dizziness, and memory problems. It can harm the health of dry-cleaning workers and of people who live near dry-cleaning businesses. The EPA has classified it as a hazardous air contaminant, while other agencies have labeled it a likely carcinogen.

Perc now contaminates up to 25 percent of U.S. drinking water, according to a government study. Although the EPA regulates the use of perc, most states have been reluctant to adopt phase-outs. One exception is California, which declared perc a toxic chemical in 1991. In 2007 state regulators enacted the nation's first ban, and by 2023 all dry-cleaning machines in the state must be perc-free.

When you bring dry-cleaned clothing into your home, perc residues remain on the fabric fibers and contaminate your air. The good news is that less toxic alternatives to conventional dry-cleaning are emerging. One popular method, "wet-cleaning," uses water and nontoxic soaps, rather than chemicals to clean fabrics—even wool. More and more cleaners are offering either wet-cleaning or liquid carbon dioxide cleaning, which has no known risks. To find a wet cleaner, go to www.nodryclean.com or www.professionalwetcleaning. com; to find a liquid carbon dioxide cleaner go to www.findco2.com.

WHAT YOU SHOULD KNOW

- Perc is used by an estimated 85 percent of dry-cleaners worldwide. According to Greenpeace, more than 95,000 tons of the solvent are used annually by 35,000 cleaners across the United States and Canada.

- Some dry cleaners routinely add mothproofing chemicals to all wool items. These chemicals contain naphthalene, which is known to produce toxic reactions, especially in newborns.

- Perc-free cleaners may use unhealthy substitutes such as petroleum-derived hydrocarbon solvents (DF-2000, EcoSolv, and Siloxane).

3 WAYS TO MAKE A SHIFT

1. Buy clothing and other fabric items that don't require dry-cleaning. It will save you money and protect your health and the environment. Look at the labels inside your clothing; sometimes "dry clean only" is just a suggestion. You may be able to wash in cold water on a gentle cycle with low or no dryer heat.

2. If your fabric item requires dry-cleaning, take it to a place that doesn't use perc. Look for "wet-cleaning" options. (If your local dry-cleaner still uses perc, educate the owner about the risks associated with the solvent and encourage him or her to switch to a less toxic alternative.)

3. When you bring home clothes from a dry-cleaner, remove the plastic covering. Let them air out for a day, then place them in your closet.

SYNTHETIC FRAGRANCES, AIR FRESHENERS, AND AEROSOL SPRAYS

If you're buying artificially scented products for your home, chances are you are exposing yourself to chemicals that are unhealthy for you. For example, in 2007 the Natural Resources Defense Council (NRDC) found that 12 of 14 popular air freshener brands contained phthalates, which you'll recall are chemicals that can cause hormonal abnormalities, birth defects, and reproductive problems.

When you see the word "fragrance" in an ingredient list, you can assume that it's 100 percent synthetic, not a blend of natural flower extracts. The

National Academy of Sciences (NAS) reports that "95 percent of the ingredients used to create fragrances today are synthetic compounds derived from petroleum, including benzene derivatives, aldehydes, and many other known toxins and sensitizers." What's more, "unscented" does not mean a product contains no fragrance. Ingredients intended to mask unpleasant odors, usually chemicals, do not have to be identified on product labels. Check that your fabric dryer sheets don't say "fragrance" on the label. If they do, it means that they contain synthetic chemicals.

Another thing to watch out for is aerosol sprays that contain flammable and nerve-damaging ingredients such as hexane and xylene. Aerosol sprays produce mist particles that can contain a high proportion of organic solvents that, when inhaled, enter your bloodstream and have negative health effects.

According to a 2007 study reported in the *American Journal of Respiratory and Critical Care Medicine*, in homes where aerosol sprays and air fresheners were used frequently, mothers experienced 25 percent more headaches and were 19 percent more likely to suffer from depression, while infants younger than 6 months had 30 percent more ear infections and a 22 percent higher incidence of diarrhea than those using non-spray cleaners. That's a lot of health problems easily rectified—and prevented—by the removal of aerosols!

WHAT YOU SHOULD KNOW

- Most air fresheners are made with synthetic fragrances containing phthalates.

- Essential oils are not the same thing as fragrance oils. Essential oils come from plants, while fragrance oils are artificially created and often contain synthetic chemicals.

- Potpourri that lists "fragrance" on the label mean that synthetic chemicals were used, and they should be avoided.

3 WAYS TO MAKE A SHIFT

1. Look for products with scents that are naturally derived or are plant-based or labeled as using essential oils. Make sure the word "fragrance" does not appear on the label.

2. For scented candles, try those made from soy or beeswax, and make sure their fragrance is made from essential oils.

3. To clear the air, use a nonaerosol citrus spray containing only citrus peel extracts, which are effective at dissolving airborne odors, instead of scented aerosol sprays, liquids that emit a continuous scent, and solid air fresheners.

Where to Shop

Your health food store is a great place to find natural cleaning products. Environmentally safe products include those made by Bon Ami, Ecover, Seventh Generation, BioShield, Earth Friendly, and EO Products; the latter offers a lavender-based line of cleaners.

Recipes to make environmentally safe cleansers from oven cleaners to mildew removers can be found online at:

- **Care 2 Make a Difference:** www.care2.com
- **Earth Easy:** www.eartheasy.com
- **Hydrogen Peroxide H$_2$O$_2$ Secrets:** www.h2o2-4u.com
- **Old Farmer's Almanac:** www.almanac.com (to find "Kitchen Tips and Tricks," go to www.almanac.com/food/tips.php)
- **Organized Home:** www.organizedhome.com
- **Toxics Use Reduction Institute:** www.turi.org

More information about safe cleaning products can be found at:

- **Green Home:** www.greenhome.com
- **Healthy Child Healthy World:** http://healthychild.org/
- **Household Products Database:** www.householdproducts.nlm.nih.gov (U.S. Department of Health and Human Services)
- **Kids Organics:** www.kidsorganics.com

Other Suggestions for Clearing the Air

Many Aftel, owner of Aftelier, a fragrance company based in Berkeley, California, suggests buying diffuser rings and filling them with essential oils for use as an air freshener. The rings fit on your light bulbs, which when turned on heat the oil and emit the fragrance.

Instead of using a bowl of synthetically scented potpourri, try putting a few drops of essential oil (lavender is nice) on a piece of cotton and place it in a bowl, or use sachets of dried flowers and herbs, which will provide gentle scents.

I use salt lamps in my home to maintain good air quality. A salt lamp is a chunk of salt crystal, usually mined from the Himalayas, that has been hollowed out to allow room for a light bulb or tiny candle. The heating of the salt causes it to release negative ions, which are found in sea air, in mountain air, and near water falls. They bind with airborne pollutants, making them heavier so that they fall to the ground, and therefore are unavailable to be inhaled. Indoor air, especially around electronic equipment, is very low in these ions. Salt lamps are a simple, natural alternative to an air purifier.

I first noticed that a salt lamp helped me when I was having an allergic reaction while visiting a friend who had cats in her home. She brought out her salt lamp, placed it on the table in front of me, and plugged it in. Within minutes I stopped sneezing. I now keep one in my bedroom, even though I don't have cats, because I find them to be relaxing and beautiful. They look like a large glowing orange stone, giving a lovely warm feeling to my room. I also keep one in my home office, near my computer.

Here are a couple of Web sites that offer good-quality salt lamps: www.naturalsaltcrystallamps.com and www.himalayansaltshop.com.

The Children's Health Environmental Coalition offers these additional tips for clearing the air:

- **Freshen rooms with cut flower, lavender, or essential oils.** Rather than relying on chemical-laden air fresheners, try floral scents from fresh flowers, lavender sachets, or essential oil on cotton balls.

- **Kill odor with naturally deodorizing and disinfecting white vinegar.** A simple recipe of 1 teaspoon baking soda, 1 teaspoon lemon juice, and 2 cups hot water in a spray bottle also works well.

- **Use baking soda or zeolite to absorb odors.** Baking soda is good for freshening musty carpets. Just sprinkle the baking soda on the carpet, let sit for a while, then vacuum. Like baking soda, the mineral zeolite can absorb odors in the air. Zeolite can be found in health food stores or online.

NONSTICK COOKWARE

The next time you find yourself standing in front of your stove, about to make a meal, think twice about using that nonstick pan. A surprising source of air pollution in the kitchen is nonstick pots and pans. When heated, they don't give off an odor, so you may not think they are a problem. But they can be.

I know they make cooking easier, but they are not so easy on your body. In just 2 or 3 minutes of preheating, your pan will give off fumes that can make you sick. Each time you use medium to high heat on an empty pan, the surface on Teflon-coated and most other nonstick cookware breaks apart and emits a toxic chemical called PFOA (perfluorooctanoic acid). Animal studies strongly suggest that when enough PFOA builds up in the body, it can cause cancer, liver damage, growth defects, and immune system damage.

While DuPont, the maker of Teflon, states that PFOA is used only in the manufacturing process and shouldn't be found in the final products, keep in mind that PFOA is a pervasive pollutant. In 2007, researchers at Johns Hopkins University analyzed nearly 300 umbilical cord blood samples and found that PFOA was detected in 99% of them. PFOA has been detected at low levels in blood bank samples in several US cities. No one knows how this chemical got into the bodies of so many people, and no one knows how severe the adverse health effects will be. What is known is that the EPA has identified PFOA as a "likely" human carcinogen, and it's clear we should be protecting ourselves and our families.

Recent studies by DuPont show that at high temperatures (over 500°F), Teflon and other similar nonstick coatings release at least six toxic gases, including two carcinogens, two global pollutants, and MFA (monofluoroacetic acid), a chemical lethal to humans at low doses. However, the Environmental Working Group warns that the coatings break down at just 325°F, or at a medium flame. Moreover, Teflon is one of the hardiest human-made products around; its molecules can survive forever in the environment and in your body. Though DuPont has never acknowledged the health dangers of PFOA exposure, the company has reduced its use in product lines by 97 percent. The company also announced in 2006 that it will phase out PFOA by 2015.

As a result of this new data, the EWG has petitioned the Consumer Product Safety Commission to require that cookware and heated appliances with nonstick coatings carry a warning label. So far, the government has not assessed the safety of nonstick cookware, and therefore there are no warning labels. In the meantime, a number of lawsuits against DuPont are pending. DuPont has been heavily fined by the EPA for allegedly hiding data for years on the toxicity of PFOA, and also for contaminating the Ohio River drinking-water supply near its West Virginia plant.

By the way, DuPont isn't the only product line that contains PFOA. Other brands include Stainmaster, Scotchgard, SilverStone, Fluron, Supra, Excalibur,

Greblon, Xylon, Duracote, Resistal, Autograph, and T-Fal. If you're thinking about Calphalon, be aware that although the nonstick coating used in Simply Calphalon cookware is not Teflon, it is made by Exxon-Mobil with the same chemical compound as Teflon.

Avian veterinarians have known for decades that Teflon off-gasses are a leading cause of death among birds, with estimates that hundreds if not thousands of birds are killed each year. Like the proverbial canary in the coal mine, birds are sensitive to their environment and act as early warning systems for humans. The EPA is recommending that bird owners completely avoid cookware and heated appliances with nonstick coatings. Perhaps humans should be heeding this warning as well!

WHAT YOU SHOULD KNOW

- PFOA is used in food packaging as a coating to prevent food from sticking to a variety of fast-food packages, including pizza boxes, microwave popcorn packages, French fry containers, and candy.

- The FDA has looked at microwaveable popcorn packaging and found that PFOA not only is present but also migrates into the oil from the packaging during heating.

- There is currently no way for you to tell whether food containers (other than glass and metal) contain PFOA.

- In 2008, the California Assembly approved a bill to ban PFOA in food containers, but then Governor Schwarzenegger vetoed the bill.

3 WAYS TO MAKE A SHIFT

1. Toss the Teflon. If you can't bring yourself to throw out every piece of nonstick-coated cookware in your kitchen, at least manage your use of it by making sure your kitchen is well-ventilated when you're cooking. Also do the following:

   - Never preheat on high or leave nonstick pans unattended over an open flame or another heat source.

   - Don't use metal utensils that can scratch the coating and release PFOA into your food.

   - Wash treated cookware by hand using nonabrasive cleaners and sponges (no steel wool). Also, avoid stacking pots and pans on top of each other; it can cause them to scratch and release the coating into your food.

2. Check out the new nontoxic nonstick cookware lines. Cuisinart has come out with its Green Gourmet line of nontoxic nonstick cookware. Martha Stewart and Green Pan Cookware have a zero–PFOA/PTFE (polytetra-fluoroethylene) (which means safe) nonstick line that uses a Thermalon coating (based on silica, which is derived from sand).

3. Consider alternatives to nonstick.

- Most chefs agree that stainless steel browns foods better than nonstick surfaces. Play around with the timing of preheating, the intensity of the flame, and amount of oil. Try using organic nonstick cooking spray.

- Cast iron is extremely durable and can now be purchased pre-seasoned and ready-to-use.

- Ceramic titanium and porcelain enameled cast iron are very durable, better at browning foods than nonstick coatings, and dishwasher safe.

- Anodized aluminum is another choice, but some people question its safety, citing evidence in studies linking aluminum exposure to Alzheimer's disease.

LEAD GLAZES IN DISHWARE

Lead, found in glazes on dishware, is a toxic substance that accumulates in your body, so even small amounts can pose a health hazard over time. According to the California Department of Health Services, lead in tableware can be a serious health threat. Some dishes contain enough lead to cause severe lead poisoning. Even dishes with lower lead levels may contribute to a person's overall lead exposure.

Since there are many thousands of different makes and kinds of china, no one has tested them all. The Environmental Defense Fund (EDF) says that really dangerous pieces of china are fairly rare, but some types of dishes are more likely to have lead. The EDF says to watch for:

- China handed down from a previous generation or found in antique stores and flea markets. These were made before lead was recognized as a hazard.

- Home-made or handcrafted china, either from the United States or abroad, unless you are sure the maker used a lead-free glaze.

Red Hot Countertops

There have been reports that some granite countertops contain high levels of uranium, which not only is radioactive but also releases radon gas as it decays. Since there is no known safe level of radon or radiation, any exposure could be a health risk.

Research scientists at Rice University in Houston and at the New York State Department of Health are conducting studies of granite used in kitchen counters.

To find a certified technician to determine whether radiation or radon is coming from your granite countertop, contact the American Association of Radon Scientists and Technologists (www.aarst.org). Also, do-it-yourself radon testing kit information is available from the EPA (www.epa.gov/radon) as well as at hardware stores and online.

One really beautiful option is to use 100% recycled glass from Ice Stone: www.icestone.biz.

- Traditional glazed terra cotta ware made in some Latin American countries, such as Mexican bean pots, unless they are specifically labeled as lead-free.

- Bright colors or decorations inside surfaces that touch the food or drink, including the rim.

- Decorations on top of the glaze instead of beneath it. If you can feel the decoration when you rub your fingers over it, or see brush strokes above the glaze surface, steer clear.

- Decoration that has begun to wear away or corrode, or one that has a dusty or chalky grey residue on the glaze after the piece has been washed. This can be dangerous and should not be used!

3 WAYS TO MAKE A SHIFT

1. Don't store food or drink in questionable china. The longer food remains in contact with a china surface containing lead, the more lead can be drawn into the food.

2. Don't serve highly acidic food or drink in questionable china. This includes cola-type soft drinks; orange and grapefruit juice; applesauce and

apple juice; tomatoes and tomato-based products, such as ketchup and spaghetti sauce; salad dressings with vinegar; and tea and coffee.

3. Don't heat or microwave in questionable china. Heat can speed up the lead-leaching process.

Many experts believe that white china is less likely to have lead problems than highly decorated, multicolored china. New china made by a well-known brand-name manufacturer is unlikely to show very high lead-leaching. However, if you are concerned, the only way to be certain is to use glass dishes without decoration, buy dishes labeled "lead-free," or do a home lead test on your existing dishes. Test kits, costing approximately $20 to $30 apiece, are available by mail and in most hardware and paint stores. They will detect only relatively high lead-leaching potential.

For more information go to the Environmental Defense Fund Web site: www.edf.org.

I know I covered a lot in this chapter and it may seem overwhelming. To make it simple, choose just one "healthy" cleaning product you can buy today and commit yourself to buying it; switch to one nonscented item, whether it's a box of garbage bags or a bag of your cat's litter; throw away one nonstick pan and replace it with a stainless steel one. These small, simple acts could have a big effect on your family's health.

UNSUNG HEROES

You probably haven't heard much about **Susan and Brad Black** and their company EO Products (EO stands for Essential Oils). That's because they've relied on word of mouth from their customers instead of advertising to get business. They started EO back in 1992, in their northern California garage. Today, it's still an independently run family company with about 30 employees.

Susan and Brad personally select every ingredient for their green business. Every certified organic formula is created from scratch for more than 100 different products for the body and home. Their vision: to make high-quality, essential oil–based products that are simple, fresh, and clean, using as many local, organic, and plant-based ingredients as possible.

In addition to their skin care products, including their popular French lavender hand soap and organic non–genetically modified organism hand sanitizer, they make truly amazing household cleaners called Greenwood Naturals. What sets it apart from other cleaners is that it is made from organic,

Are You Chemically Sensitive?

Airborne chemicals can make people feel ill. More and more people are becoming sensitive to fragrances, including perfumes or scented household and cleaning products. Manufacturers are adding scents to things such as garbage bags, kitty litter, and baby wipes. If you experience such symptoms as headaches, dizziness, or breathing difficulties, you may have an environmentally triggered condition called multiple chemical sensitivity (MCS). In serious cases it can lead to devastating fatigue.

Chemical sensitivities are very much based on the individual. In other words, no one can tell you exactly how much of chemical X is just enough to cause serious harm in you. It may do little to your friend, but wreak havoc in your body. Everyone has a unique chemical "threshold," so to speak, above which a certain chemical goes from relatively harmless to highly dangerous. Studies done on products to determine their level of "safety" are general, and by no means do they reflect what's safe for every individual.

In addition, toxic chemicals can react in unexpected ways, especially when combined with other chemicals. And the factors that trigger illness and disease in any given individual are, to a large extent, vague and unknown. It's estimated that 25 to 45 million people in the United States have some type of chemical sensitivity.

If you have MCS, think of yourself as a canary of the 21st century. Canaries were used by miners during the 1700s to detect methane gas and in the 1900s to detect carbon monoxide. The birds would faint or die before the miners would notice the dangerous gases. Today, chemically sensitive people might just be detecting toxic stuff in the environment before others are able to. Just because some of us can't smell it doesn't mean volatile organic compounds (VOCs) are not affecting us. In one study, Gary Schwartz, PhD, and his research team at the University of Arizona showed that the brain registers exposure to a chemical odor even though the nose does not sense its presence.

wild-crafted raw materials that envelop you in the soothing scent of actual lavender hydrosol and essential oil. Greenwood Naturals products are the result of volunteer efforts of parents at the Greenwood School in Mill Valley, California. A portion of profits from the sale of these household cleaners goes to the Greenwood School tuition-assistance fund.

The Greenwood Naturals line consists of three items: All Purpose Cleaner, a liquid concentrate that will clean your floors, car, and anything else dirty; the Countertop Spray, which handles fingerprints, spattered grease, even ants (when you run out, add a ¼ cup All Purpose Cleaner to a bottle of water, and you've got a refill); and the Dishsoap, which cleans your dishes with real lavender hydrosol and essential oil, not a fabricated lavender "fragrance." All are biodegradable and completely nontoxic. You can purchase Greenwood Naturals as well as other EO products at selected retail stores or on the company Web site: www. eoproducts.com.

For the latest eco-cleaning products, visit: www.supernaturalhome.com.

Chapter 10

SUPER NATURAL HOME AWAY FROM HOME

How to Maintain Your New Lifestyle on the Road, at Work, at School, and at Play

"As a child my family's menu consisted of two choices: take it or leave it."

—BUDDY HACKETT

NOW THAT YOU'VE BECOME MORE AWARE of your exposure to toxins in your home, and you've done what you can to eliminate or reduce them, it's time to pay attention to the choices you make outside of your home. There are lots of them, from the food you get in restaurants, vending machines, and school or work cafeterias to the summer camps your kids attend and the hotels you stay in. Every day, with even the smallest or most mundane transactions, you make choices that can enhance your well-being, improve your health, and help the planet. Remember, all products that are toxic to us are also toxic to the planet because when we discard them their chemicals return into the air, water, and soil.

What I do is try to choose products that come from nature instead of a chemical factory. For example, I will buy a cotton shirt over one made of polyester, or a beeswax or soy candle instead of one made from paraffin, a petroleum derivative. Another thing I like to do is think about whether I can see the sun in what I buy. Fruits and vegetables? Easy. Food-like products that come in a box? Not so easy. Grass-fed beef, chicken, and eggs? Easy. Energy bars? Not so easy. You can even see the sun in the paper in this book, if you use your imagination. Think about it—it was necessary for the sun to shine on the trees, which were then harvested and eventually turned into paper.

I also consider whether each product I buy is in harmony with nature and supports life on Earth—in other words, how "green" it is. Consumer advocate Debra Lynn Dadd defines green as something that "supports, enhances and celebrates life." In her book *Really Green* she points out that there is no legal definition of "green," nor is there a regulatory definition. But the one question you can ask yourself each time you reach for a product is, does it sustain life or not? "A green product does more good than harm," Dadd says.

I discovered a good green product while shopping for a throw rug for my daughter's bedroom. Instead of buying one made from synthetic materials manufactured in a factory, we found a lovely fuzzy, purple one made from wool, which is a renewable resource (the sheep enjoy being sheared, especially in the summer!), and dyed by using natural vegetable dyes. The rug, by Flokati, was hand woven the way it has been for centuries in Greece. There was a story about the origin of the rugs on display at the store where it was sold. These rugs originally served as bedding to keep shepherds warm in their tents during the winter. After they are woven, they are placed on rocks under the Pindos Mountains' waterfalls for 40 hours. There their backings swell and their pile unravels and fluffs. Each rug is then hung to dry in the Greek sun.

OK, so after I read this amazing story, I just *had* to buy one of the rugs. I was expecting it to be very expensive, but relatively speaking, it wasn't. It cost $71, about twice that of a synthetic one, but I knew the rug wouldn't off-gas or make my daughter's feet itch. And it was machine washable! It's a rug my grandmother would have been proud to have in her home as well. I found it at my local green store, Green Fusion Design Center in San Anselmo, California (www.greenfusiondesigncenter.com); it's also sold at Pottery Barn Teens (www.pbteens.com).

Here are some other ways to take your Super Natural Home consciousness with you when you shop.

SHOPPING WITH CONSCIOUSNESS

Lynne Twist writes in her book *The Soul of Money* that when her first grand-child was born, she couldn't wait to go shopping for her. She planned a big day at the mall, but just before she left her house, she got a call from her son, the baby's father, encouraging her to purchase things "that are produced and made in ways we feel good about." He wanted Lynne to buy only from those stores or brands that represent natural, sustainable manufacturing and fair labor practices. In addition, he kindly but firmly asked Lynne to not buy the baby more than she needed because he didn't want to begin a pattern of excess.

Lynne remembers being totally shocked by the conversation. "His words didn't match the picture of the shopping spree that had filled my mind," she recalls. As a social activist, Lynne was working to stop child labor in developing countries and helping to clean up the environment, yet, she says, she "was completely blind to the fact that I was ready to buy anything and everything for my adorable granddaughter, with no consciousness about where it came from, who made it, how it was made, and any consequences that came from that."

Lynne's story illustrates how easy it is to get caught up in the impulse to buy, to get sucked in by marketing tactics and cultural pressure. She decided to honor her son's request and shopped with consciousness. She read labels, asked questions, learned about fabrics and origins of materials, and felt good about buying items from companies and craftspeople who shared her values.

Lynne teaches a good lesson that we can apply when we shop. Follow her advice and look at labels, ask questions, and learn about the origins of the products you buy. This is especially important when shopping for food. You may feel powerless when it comes to buying food because you think that your choices for healthy food are limited. But know that the food industry takes its cues from shoppers. "If you walk into Wal-Mart or Whole Foods and exercise a vote for organic, local, or climate-friendly, you can change the world," says Gary Hirshberg, CEO of Stonyfield Farm organic yogurt.

To take this a step further, ask your local market to stock organic food (as well as nontoxic cleaners) if they don't. "The fact that customers are interested and making their preferences known—that alone moves and shapes the world," Gary says.

3 WAYS TO MAKE A SHIFT

1. Choose products that come from nature. (Can you see the sun in it?)
2. Bring consciousness to every purchase you make.
3. Buy only what you need.

EATING OUT

When you go to a restaurant, there are easy things you can do to eat with consciousness—the way you've started to if you've been following the suggestions in this book. First, remember to ask for what you want, even if it's not on the menu. Most restaurants will gladly prepare a vegetarian entrée for you, or steamed vegetables instead of fried. Ask for the sauce (which probably contains lots fat and sugar) on the side instead of poured over your meat or fish or veggies. Ask if the fish is wild or farm raised; ask if the chickens are free range and whether the beef was grass fed. If enough people do this, restaurants may start offering more of what you want.

Ask the restaurant manager what type of oil they use for frying. Chances are it is partially hydrogenated vegetable oil. Ask if they'd consider switching to, for example, rice bran oil. This oil costs about the same as vegetable oil; has a very high smoke (burn) point, making it perfect for deep frying or pan or stir frying; and contains no trans-fatty acids, since hydrogenation isn't required for its stability. Tell them that "hydrogenated vegetable oil is a toxic substance that does not belong in food," according to Walter Willett, MD, chair of the department of nutrition at the Harvard School of Public Health.

The Center for Science in the Public Interest has called for city, state, and federal governments to take action to completely eliminate trans fats from our food. Slowly, cities across America are heeding the call. Tiburon, California; New York City and nearby Westchester County, New York; Boston; Philadelphia; Seattle; and Baltimore are among the first to ban trans fats in restaurants. Los Angeles is considering the ban; Los Angeles County has implemented a voluntary program in which restaurants can be certified as "trans fat free" and receive a decal to display that fact to customers. Now, California has become the first state in the nation to require menu labeling at chain restaurants. Other states will sure to follow.

3 WAYS TO MAKE A SHIFT

1. Ask for what you want, even if it's not on the menu.
2. Avoid food that is deep fried (that includes donuts); it most probably contains trans fats.
3. Ask your local restaurants to switch to rice bran oil or another oil that contains no trans fats.

EATING AT THE OFFICE

At work, forgo the donuts at staff meetings and make a request for fresh fruit or pastries that don't contain a lot of fat or sugar. If coffee is provided at work, ask your employer to purchase an organic and fair trade brand. Use your own reusable cups instead of drinking from plastic or Styrofoam. Ask your employer to install a water filtration system or water cooler that uses natural spring water.

3 WAYS TO MAKE A SHIFT

1. Opt for fresh fruit at meetings.
2. Request organic and fair trade coffee.
3. Request a water filtration system or cooler.

EATING ON THE ROAD

If you've ever traveled for work, you're well aware that there's no good food on planes or at most hotels catering to business travelers. The best thing to do is carry food onto the plane so you won't have to rely on the airport food kiosks or in-flight meals. I always pack satisfying snacks such as crackers and cheese, raw nuts, fresh and dried fruit, or a healthy sandwich when I fly.

Checking into a hotel often means checking your Super Natural Home consciousness at the door. But it doesn't have to. One friend of mine who travels a lot for business says she prefers using room service so that she can relax in her room instead of eating alone in the hotel's restaurant. But there's a caveat: "I always tell them what I want, and never order off the menu," she says. She

Happy at Work

For happier employees, grow plants at the office, suggests a February 2008 study by the American Society for Horticultural Science. Workers who spend longer hours under artificial light in windowless offices report reduced job satisfaction and increased stress levels. The answer? Have live plants or a view of the outside.

The organization Green Plants for Green Buildings recommends placing one plant per every 100 square feet. If you're interested in boosting productivity and just feeling better while working in your office, try adding a few of the plants listed in Chapter 8.

---

usually orders a baked potato and steamed vegetables. "I ask for some type of green vegetable even though it's not listed on the menu, and they always give it to me," she adds. She also takes her own healthy snacks to avoid raiding the mini-bar.

Even traveling for pleasure can be challenging when it comes to eating healthy. One winter my family and I went skiing in Copper Mountain, Colorado, and I made the wrong assumption that we would find some healthy food options at the ski village. Boy, was I wrong! There was one small market, and I couldn't find anything remotely healthy to eat except some mushy apples and wilted lettuce. Even the peanut butter had hydrogenated oil and sugar in it. Almost all the restaurants served "bar food," which was basically deep-fried fare. I wound up eating what was available, but in the future I will pack some basic snacks like organic peanut butter, crackers, and some raw nuts and seeds.

Another ski trip, this time to Squaw Valley, California, presented a different kind of food issue. We found a lovely restaurant that featured organic and local food, and our daughter, then 7 years old, ordered the macaroni and cheese from their kids' menu.

When her food came, I was shocked to see that such an upscale organic restaurant would serve macaroni and cheese that looked like it came right out of a box from a popular brand notorious for their artificial ingredients. Included was apple sauce, served in a small round plastic cup, that was clearly a mass-produced item as well. When I asked the waiter, he told me these were indeed products from a major manufacturer. That company had a deal with the resort to supply all the kids' meals on the slopes—even at this restaurant.

I spoke with the manager, who told me that "kids have a different type of palette than adults and prefer this type of food." I told him how disappointed I was that their chef couldn't at least use an organic pasta and cheese recipe. He told me he would make the request to the chef. I haven't been back to this restaurant, but in the future, at other restaurants, I will ask if the kids' menu is prepared with the same food as the adult menu.

3 WAYS TO MAKE A SHIFT

1. Pack your own food and snacks for your trip. Try bringing some sort of superfoods green powder (sold in natural foods markets). Just add water to create an instant meal; shake it up in a bottle or blend it with a mini hand-held mixer. Or pack organic food bars and don't rely on vending machines.

2. When using room service, ask for what you want even if you don't see it on the menu. Seek out the healthiest foods you can find.

3. Don't forget to pack your own personal care products, so you don't have to rely on the shampoo and soap in the hotel.

PACKING FOR THE PLANE

In addition to carrying my own food on board, for trips longer than 5 hours I always take a product called No Jet Lag, a homeopathic remedy made into in small pellets that dissolve in your mouth. I find it has no side effects and works wonderfully, even for long flights abroad. No Jet Lag can be found at Whole Foods, the Vitamin Shoppe, and some pharmacies.

I also use Airborne, a top-selling dietary supplement that boosts the body's immune system by supplying it with an assortment of vitamins, minerals, and herbs. In June 2008, Airborne settled a class action lawsuit that challenged the company's advertising and labeling claims. However, this shouldn't deter you. In an informal survey of flight attendants on United and Southwest airlines, almost everyone I asked uses Airborne on a regular basis. Also, friends of mine who travel frequently won't leave home without it. They dissolve the effervescent tablet (like Alka-Seltzer) in water and drink it every couple of hours on a flight. Airborne can be found at your

"I never eat airline food."

—Peter Greenberg, travel editor, the *Today* show

local drugstore (Walgreens has its own knock-off version) and at many supermarkets. Make sure you choose the flavor that contains no aspartame!

I also fill a small spray bottle with purified water and citrus essential oils and spritz my face during flights to avoid getting sick. A friend of mine takes a lemon on board and scores it with a knife (plastic of course!) and inhales the vapors. Since lemons are antibacterial, he says this technique has prevented him from getting sick when he travels. Another friend of mine, who has flown over 1 million miles, swears by this old-fashioned technique: He sprinkles a few drops each of lavender, peppermint, and lemon essential oils onto a silk handkerchief and sniffs it during the flight. He says he's never been sick either. You can find silk handkerchiefs in most men's stores.

You might want to consider using a personal or miniature air purifier to minimize your exposure to toxins such as the fumes in the recirculated air from lubricating oils, deicing fluids, and other industrial pollutants from normal plane operations; volatile organic compounds that come from cleaning products and cabin materials; and infectious agents that come from passengers. The Ultra-Miniature Air Supply costs about $150, and its manufacturer, Wein Products, claims it is "the world's first wearable air purifier." According to their Web site (www.weinproducts.com), tests at UCLA School of Microbiology resulted in a "90% reduction in germ colony growth." They say the Good Housekeeping Institute tested it against cat allergen and cigarette smoke and recommended it. You will often see it advertised in in-flight shopping catalogs, and you can order directly from the Wein Web site.

Another idea given to me by a trusted frequent-flyer friend is to sleep in a silk bed sack when traveling. Silk is a naturally hypoallergenic material that is inhospitable to dust mites and resists moisture, mildew, and odors. It acts as a barrier for allergy-sensitive skin from unfamiliar hotel or motel bedding and protects you from both germs and harsh chemicals used in laundering. It's great for sleeping on the plane, too. You can find silk bed sacks online at: www.amazon.com and www.allergybuyersclubshopping.com.

When flying, be sure to drink plenty of water—and not the water from the tap on the plane. Ask for bottled spring water, if available.

GREEN TRAVEL AND VACATION

Green travel is still in its infancy, but as eco-hotels go from thatched-roof bungalows in the jungle to more mainstream, there are more and more options to choose from. Many hotels are now offering more than just energy-saving options as part of their green initiative to help the planet. Some hotels provide items such as natural bath products and organic food. For example, Kimpton Hotels uses nontoxic, citrus-based cleaners as well as organic amenities in their guest rooms. Fairmont Hotels and InterContinental are renovating with eco-friendly building materials.

San Francisco's Hotel Triton has decorated a room on each floor using environmentally safe paints, furniture created from salvaged forest-fire wood, and organic hemp towels and sheets. Las Vegas, usually known for excess, could soon be home to the world's largest concentration of environmentally friendly hotel rooms. Fifteen major new building projects, including the MGM Mirage's new 4,000-room CityCenter (set to open in late 2009), are seeking the building council's stringent Leadership in Environment and Energy Design (LEED) Certification.

One thing to do before you book a hotel room is to ask if the hotel policy is to avoid harsh chemicals, such as scented laundry supplies, carpet cleaners, and air fresheners. I've been to a five-star hotel that used such strong-smelling cleaners I requested my room be aired out before I used it.

For help in finding a green, eco-friendly hotel, go to the Green Hotels Association Web site, www.greenhotels.com, for a current listing of hotel members. The online travel site Orbitz (www.orbitz.com) also offers environmentally friendly hotel packages. The following Web sites may be helpful:

- www.environmentallyfriendlyhotels.com, which offers reviews of green lodgings
- www.gobeyondgreen.org, the latest in environmentally friendly and eco-progressive travel
- www.greenglobetrotter.blogspot.com, blog full of great info and resources

Spa Treatments and Facials

Find out which skin care products spas use before you book your service. Ask if the products contain parabens or artificial colors or other irritants. Check out the resource directory www.spafinder.com, which lists spas that offer healing traditions and ingredients from the local culture.

Insect Repellent

Every year, approximately one-third of the U.S. population uses insect repellants containing DEET to ward off mosquitoes and other pests. At present, DEET is an ingredient in more than 230 products, with concentrations of up to 100 percent. Duke University Medical Center pharmacologist Mohamed Abou-Donia, PhD, who has spent 30 years researching the effects of pesticides, discovered that prolonged exposure to DEET can damage brain cells. When rats had their skin treated with the average human dosage equivalent (40 mg/kg body weight) of DEET for 60 days, they performed far worse than control rats on physical tests requiring muscle control, strength, and coordination. They also had a harder time accomplishing easy tasks such as walking.

Natural alternatives to DEET-containing insect repellents include the following (these can be found in natural food stores, in some pharmacies, and online where indicated):

- Aubrey, Gone!
- Badger Balm, Anti-Bug Formula
- Bug Off! By SunFeather Natural Soap Company (www.sunfeather.com)
- Califonia Baby Bug Repellent Spray
- Dr. Mercola's Bug Off (www.mercola.com)
- Kiss My Face, Swy Flotter
- Repel, Plant Based Insect Repellent

You also might try making your own insect repellent. Here's an easy recipe* that requires only a spray bottle, a funnel, and the following ingredients:

⅓ cup of apple cider vinegar

⅓ cup witch hazel (or inexpensive vodka)

5 drops of citronella or eucalyptus essential oil

Using the funnel, pour all the liquid ingredients into the spray bottle. Shake to mix the liquids.

You're now holding a bottle of effective, organic bug repellent. Unlike the store-bought sprays, this isn't waterproof (or sweat-proof), so reapply as necessary.

*Source: DIY Network (www.diynetwork.com)

- www.itsagreengreenworld.com, a global listing of eco-friendly hospitality destinations
- www.sustainabletravelinternational.org, information on eco-travel

EATING AT SCHOOL

In school cafeterias, unhealthy foods and drinks—highly processed and packaged, often sweetened with high-fructose corn syrup—are the rule rather than the exception. This is not the sort of diet that can help a child's brain and body develop optimally.

Given the high rate of obesity among our children, coupled with the growing demand on our health care system, there's never been a better time to instigate changes in how our school systems buy, prepare, and serve food to our kids. The percentage of overweight children in the United States is increasing at an alarming rate, with one out of three kids now considered overweight or obese. Children and teens spend a great deal of their time in school. Helping them develop healthy habits early on will benefit everyone, including childless adults. After all, top health officials looking to reform health care for everyone in America have stated over and over again that the revolution must start with the younger generation. The sooner we can lower all the risk factors for disease that accompany being overweight, the sooner we can establish a stronger and more accessible health care system.

Several years ago, I, along with five other moms from different private schools in my area, initiated the first organic hot lunch program at our schools. The process took a full year; even in Marin County, home to the organic food movement, I met with resistance. First, I sent out a survey to parents asking if they'd be interested in having their children receive organic lunches and if they'd be willing to pay one or two dollars more per day than what they were paying for corn dogs, canned fruit, and chips (a common meal). I received comments like "My child won't eat bean sprouts!" or "My child likes to eat *tasty* food!" I had to explain that organic didn't mean either of those. It just meant there would be no pesticides or genetically modified organisms in our children's meals. After we got the go-ahead from the parents and heads of schools, we interviewed a series of caterers and local organic markets. One called The Good Earth in Fairfax, California, won—their food passed the taste test (we had kids sample the food), and they were less expensive than the caterers. The Good Earth hired a chef and rented a facility to accommodate

Another great thing to do at school is to use no-waste lunches. This involves a reusable lunch box, waxed paper instead of plastic, recycled aluminum foil, cloth napkins, and a metal water bottle. Make sure you offer organic food, including snacks, in those lunch boxes! One place to buy a reusable, waste-free lunch kit is www.kidskonserve.com.

our needs, since this was their first venture into a large-scale lunch program. It was agreed that the food would look and taste as similar to the food the kids were already getting in their current hot lunch program, only healthier (no corn dogs!).

Since they didn't make pizza the way the kids were used to seeing it, they contracted with a local pizza parlor and supplied them with organic whole wheat pizza dough. I watched with anticipation that first day the new, organic pizza was delivered. And you know what? The kids hated it! They wouldn't eat it. It was too dry, they said. So a compromise was reached; from then on, all the pizza, bread and pasta would be made from organic *white* flour instead of whole wheat.

The challenges continued. I was also on a committee to plan a school picnic. The majority of the parents on the committee voted for hot dogs, pizza, and watermelon. I raised my hand and asked if it would be possible to have organic food at the event. The chair of the committee said, "No, we're just going to have *normal* food." I countered with, "So by normal, you mean food that's been sprayed with pesticides?" There was silence. Then I asked if we could at least have organic watermelon. "What are you . . . a food Nazi?" the chairperson asked. (It's hard to believe that this conversation took place in Marin County!) This time the silence came from me. I decided to ignore her question and volunteered to call one of the local farms and have organic watermelons delivered to our picnic.

Currently, the organic hot lunch program is running smoothly, and The Good Earth now services 11 other private schools in Marin County. Admittedly, it may be easier to get a program going at a private school than at a public school offering a low-cost or free lunch program because of the bureaucratic approval process involved. But did you know that both the Physicians Committee for Responsible Medicine and the Healthy School Lunch Campaign say that the "menus served in school lunch programs are too rich in saturated fat and cholesterol and too low in fiber- and nutrient-rich fruits, vegetables, whole grains, and legumes"?

It's up to us to ask our school boards to make healthy changes in the meals and snacks that include less sugar; fewer trans fats and less high-fructose corn syrup; and more fresh foods, whole grains, and organic or local ingredients. It's a movement that should encompass all schools, including preschools, daycare operations, Sunday schools, and colleges and universities. Think about the transformation that can occur if we had fewer cases of obesity and diabetes!

An example of this sort of positive change is the founding of the nonprofit Edible Schoolyard in Berkeley, California, by Alice Waters, famed chef, cookbook author, and owner of the restaurant Chez Panisse. Waters launched the Edible Schoolyard in 1994, and within 2 years, she transformed asphalt schoolyards into organic gardens where kids learn about food and their connection to nature. In the garden, students are involved in all aspects of planting and cultivation; in the kitchen-classroom, they prepare, serve, and eat food, some of which they have grown themselves. These activities are woven into the curriculum and are part of the school day. To find out how to start a garden at your child's school, visit www.edibleschoolyard.org.

Another solution taking root across America is the Farm to School program. It educates kids about local food by organizing field trips to small local farms and providing health and nutrition education that will hopefully influence their food choices for a lifetime. In addition to farm visits, schools buy and serve foods such as organic fruits and vegetables, and local eggs, honey, meat, and beans. They also incorporate nutrition-based curriculum and

School Lunch/Snack Ideas

- Red bell pepper strips and carrot sticks (my grade-school–age daughter will eat carrots if I serve them with the green tops, Bugs Bunny–style)
- Smoothies (put them in a thermos or drink bottle)
- Roll-ups or pita pockets with cheese (plus other toppings, like lettuce or avocado, if your child will eat them)

- Cut-up fruit, vegetables, or cheese on a stick
- Colorful fruit salad
- Homemade muffins
- Quesadillas, made with melted cheese on a whole-wheat or corn tortilla
- Homemade soup (put in a wide-mouthed thermos)

provide students with experiential learning about gardening, recycling, and sustainable agriculture. It's a win-win: kids gain a whole new perspective on food, and farmers have access to a new market. To learn more, go to www. farmtoschool.org.

Good Reasons to Have a Garden and a Kitchen at Your Child's School

- Students understand the role of food in life, as well as improving nutrition and highlighting healthy foods.
- Students learn about where food really comes from and about seasonality, life cycles, rituals, and celebrations.
- These programs provide opportunities for community involvement, establishing a link with neighbors, volunteers, parents, and community businesses.
- They also teach students life skills such as gardening and cooking.

How to Create an Organic School Lunch Program at Your Child's School

1. Familiarize yourself with your school district's policy regarding meals and snacks sold in school stores and/or vending machines.
2. Eat a typical lunch at the school if possible. Consult the curriculum, the teachers, or the school health staff to determine if students receive any instruction in nutrition and healthy eating. Talk with food service workers to get their opinions on what students do and don't eat.
3. Discuss your concerns with your school's decision makers:
   - the school food services director
   - the principal
   - the PTO/PTA
   - school board members
4. Organize a committee. Enlist parents, teachers, and staff to join.
5. Recruit helpful community members, such as a pediatrician, nurse, or nutrition expert. Identify students to serve on your committee or help with the project. Student participation is key!

6. Know the reason for organics at schools. Use the information from the following sources to build your case and become informed:

- All Organic Links page: www.allorganiclinks.com
- Beyond Pesticides: www.beyondpesticides.org
- The Eat Well Guide: www.eatwellguide.com
- Fresh Baby: www.freshbaby.com
- Generation Green: www.generationgreen.org
- National Farm to School: www.farmtoschool.org
- Organic Valley: www.organicvalley.com
- Organic.org: www.organic.org
- Organics Consumers Association: www.organicconsumers.org
- Stonyfield Farm: www.stonyfield.com
- If you have a co-op in your area, you may want to contact them for additional resources.)

7. Involve the media. Write letters to the editor about the problems you see and ways that you feel they can be corrected. Cite statistics. Send press releases to local newspapers and radio stations to announce events or

(continued on page 184)

Artificial Turf and Lead at School

In May 2008, the US Environmental Protection Agency decided to investigate whether synthetic playing fields can be hazardous when inhaled and whether the fake blades of grass contain unsafe lead levels. When the synthetic surface (made from nylon and rubber granules) heats up, it emits gases known as polycyclic aromatic hydrocarbons (PAHs), which could be carcinogenic, according to international studies.

It is recommended that you ask the managers of your local playing field what kind of turf they use and suggest testing if they don't know what it's made of. If high lead levels are suspected, the field should be wet down before use to depress dust levels, says Eddy Bresnitz, MD, epidemiologist for the State of New Jersey. "After playing on the field, people, particularly children, should wash their hands and faces, and remove their clothing to avoid inhaling or ingesting contaminants," he adds.

Hospitals with Heart

If you've ever been a patient or visited someone in a hospital, you know how unhealthy the environment can be. Take the food, for example. It could use some reconstructive surgery!

I was shocked to read the label on a "smoothie" served to a friend of mine who couldn't eat solid food after a procedure. There were over 30 ingredients, most of them artificial sweeteners and preservatives, on the list! I quickly ran out and bought a similar drink at Whole Foods that contained only fresh fruit and some protein powder; I honestly thought what the hospital was serving could impede my friend's recovery from her procedure and might possibly make her sick.

A 2003 article in the journal *Nutrition* showed that hospitalized patients worldwide are malnourished, and rates of undernourishment in some U.S. hospitals were as high as 41 percent. In 2006, a research letter in the *Journal of the American Board of Family Medicine* reported that 42 percent of large U.S. teaching hospitals had brand-name fast-food franchises right on hospital grounds. The most common fast food sold in hospitals? Krispy Kreme doughnuts.

Health Care Without Harm, a nonprofit organization, created a campaign to convince hospitals to serve more local fruits and vegetables, hormone-free milk, meat raised without antibiotics or hormones, and eggs laid by cage-free hens. Thus far, hospitals in 21 states, ranging in size from 25 to 900 beds, have signed the pledge.

After you read about the following two hospitals, it might inspire you to suggest to your local hospital to make some positive changes to their food service, or even to suggest that they try using nontoxic disinfectants to cut down on the amount of chemicals patients are exposed to.

The newly constructed Henry Ford Hospital in West Bloomfield, Illinois, outside of Chicago, is revolutionizing the way hospital food service is done. In addition to focusing on wellness and healing by offering services that include health coaches, holistic therapies, and personal trainers to help people control or prevent chronic conditions, it created an amazing dining program that uses organic and sustainably grown produce.

"Wellness starts with food," hospital president and chief executive officer Gerard van Grinsven explains. "In the old days, food was medicine. We want to go back to that idea and, through food, help our patients in healing faster and recovering faster. . . . And, we want to educate them to change their eating habits when they go back home."

What sets this hospital apart from others is that patients can order nutritious meals for delivery to their rooms 24 hours a day. The food doesn't come from a freezer or package, or from an outside vendor. It is cooked fresh using natural and organic ingredients. To help patients eat healthier once they go home, cooking classes are held in the hospital's cooking studio. Patients go there or watch on their in-room TVs.

Their meals contain no trans fats, fried foods (including french fries), or nitrates, and have more vegetables, whole-grain breads, brown rice instead of white, and only very lean meat, or chicken and turkey.

Another hospital on the right track in terms of wellness is Kaiser Permanente, the largest nonprofit health maintenance organization in the country. Starting about 5 years ago,

Kaiser opened 40 weekly organic farmers' markets for hospital staff, visitors and the community right outside their facilities all over the country. The program was started by Preston Maring, MD, one of Kaiser's doctors. He's working to create a system that sources food for inpatient meals from small family farmers as well.

In addition, following 2 and a half years of testing and research, Kaiser decided in September 2004 to lower the total chemical load people are exposed to in a hospital setting. They have moved away from using PVC in its flooring materials, including the backing used in its carpeting, and are using alternatives for items such as the tubing used in neonatal intensive care that contained DEPH—a plasticizer that is added to vinyl as a softener (listed by the National Toxicology Program as a probable human carcinogen and endocrine disruptor). Asked why the hospital created this initiative, Tom Cooper, Kaiser's manager of strategic sourcing and technology replied: "There's such a direct link between chemicals, the environment, and healthcare, that it's only natural."

important meetings. Suggest your local paper do a feature story on school lunches. If the school has a newspaper, get students to write articles on the need for organics.

8. Write letters to public officials to help change public policy. Be sure to include letters from the students.

9. Stay tuned to the process. Whether your school agrees to ban some junk foods, discontinue vending services, or change the cafeteria menu, stay involved. Keep your commitment intact to oversee the process and to step in if implementation doesn't go as expected.

10. Inspire others. Celebrate all victories no matter how small. Tell your story to the media. Share your story with others by sending an e-mail to the following:

- Beyond Pesticides at info@beyondpesticides.org
- Stonyfield's Creating Healthy Kids blog at menuforchange@stonyfield.com

Adapted from Stonyfield Farm's Menu for Change "Ten Steps to Changing Your School's Menu" (www.stonyfield.com/MenuForChange/parentsAction/MFCParentActionKit.cfm)

SUMMER CAMP FOOD CAUTION

Sending your child to sleep-away camp this summer? Be aware that the food being served might be scarier than the tales told around the campfire. Before signing up my daughter for her first adventure away from home, I logged onto the camp Web site to check out the menu. I was dismayed to see the following foods being offered: corn dogs, taquitos, fried chicken, chicken nuggets, tater tots, coffee cake, croissants, and lemonade.

I knew that these foods were laden with trans fats. Plus, the lemonade, I discovered, is made from a powdered drink mix and is made available to the kids throughout the day. Almost all powdered juice drinks are sweetened with high-fructose corn syrup, which I knew to be unhealthy. I was convinced that my daughter's health would be negatively impacted and she would surely gain weight consuming these types of foods.

I emailed the camp director with my concerns. He suggested I speak directly to the camp chef, who admitted to using partially hydrogenated vegetable oil. I asked him if he would be willing to switch to trans fat free rice oil. His reply: "While I do use rice oil at home, we feed over 600 children a week at this camp, and unless there is a law requiring me to switch, I won't change oils." I then asked him if he would consider using fresh juice or a concentrate without high-fructose corn syrup. Again he stated: "No, not unless there is a law saying I must do that."

I felt discouraged. My husband and I decided this was a deal breaker and we would search for another camp. But this story has a happy ending. The following week I got a call from the camp director, who said: "I thought seriously about what you said about nutrition and have decided to hire a new food service provider and a nutritionist. We will be using trans fat–free cooking oil, adding more fresh fruits and fewer desserts, and replacing the powdered juice drinks with real juice."

Wow! I was elated! It's proof that change starts by just asking the question. Be bold and don't be afraid to continue fighting for what you want. More than likely, you'll eventually see positive results. So what is my next step after this experience? Organically grown food. I'll make that request next summer!

UNSUNG HERO

Stephen Joseph is the founder of BanTransFats.com. He works behind the scenes on a daily basis to help the food industry reduce and eliminate trans fat in our food supply and educate the public about its harmful effects. He's also the lawyer who sued Kraft/Nabisco in 2003 to ban the marketing and sale of trans fat–laden Oreo cookies to children, and to prevent Kraft from continuing to distribute Oreo cookies to young kids in schools. As a result of the lawsuit, Kraft agreed to remove partially hydrogenated oil from Oreo cookies and reduce or eliminate it in about 650 of Kraft's other products.

Dying to be Green

If you don't want to be wrapped in plastic and preserved in embalming fluid (aka toxic chemicals) when you are buried, or release toxic mercury into the air and the land when you're cremated, you can have an environmentally sound funeral using a biodegradable coffin leaving no trace of yourself when you naturally decompose. The Natural Burial Company is the country's first biodegradable-coffin gallery, offering caskets made of handmade silk paper, wicker, and even recycled newspapers: www.natural-burialcompany.com

The Oreo lawsuit had a huge domino effect. The publicity that the lawsuit received created public awareness about the trans fat issue and triggered an avalanche of events, including a new labeling rule by the FDA. Stephen's organization also sued McDonald's in 2003 for misleading its customers into believing that it had switched to a cooking oil lower in trans fats. As a result, McDonald's agreed to inform its customers that it had not changed to the lower–trans fat cooking oil by placing prominent notices in all of its restaurants nationwide and in the media. It also agreed to pay $7 million to the American Heart Association for a trans fat program.

Stephen's organization made Tiburon, California, "America's first trans fat-free city." Project Tiburon was intended to be an inspiration and model for other towns and cities, and as a result Stephen was contacted by New York City officials, who wanted to copy the idea. New York City passed a regulation banning trans fat in December 2006. In February 2007, Philadelphia followed suit. Other cities are poised to do the same. For more information, go to www. bantransfats.com.

Epilogue

ACTION PLAN

10 Easy Ways to Have a Super Natural Home

"Knowing is not enough! You must take action."

—ANTHONY ROBBINS

GETTING TO THE END of a book like this can leave you wondering, "Okay, what am I supposed to do first?" To begin, pat yourself on the back for all that you've learned. Even if you don't remember every fact or piece of advice, chances are you have already made vast improvements in your life. Seriously! I bet you've already begun to live more consciously, without even knowing it. That's what happens when you gain new knowledge. It becomes a part of your lifestyle sooner—and more effortlessly—than you think.

Don't let this be the end. Keep this book on an accessible shelf and go back to any section or chapter at any time when you're ready to make a change in one area of your life. Remember, this is not an all-or-nothing approach, and I don't expect anyone to implement all of these ideas right away. Go at your own pace and choose those recommendations that are most suitable to your lifestyle, wallet, and psyche.

Taking one doable step at a time reminds me of an experience I had about 20 years ago when I went on an Outward Bound Wilderness trip, designed to help people discover and develop their potential through challenging endeavors in unfamiliar settings. A group of about a dozen of us were hiking in Joshua Tree National Park, when the time came to do some rock climbing. Now, I grew up in New York City and had never been to the desert, so it felt like being in the middle of nowhere. I was terrified at the thought of climbing a 100-foot rock!

One of my group mates at the base of the rock was called my belay. Belaying is the technique of controlling the rope so that a falling climber does not fall very far. The belay must be alert and ready to perform at a moment's notice; communication is extremely important. When you belay you literally hold your partner's life in your hands, which proved to be true for me that very hot morning.

As I ascended, I noticed that I easily was able to make big strides and climb up the rock fairly quickly. Then suddenly, about half way up, I stopped. The tips of my fingers were bleeding, my mouth was parched, and my knees were shaking. The temperature was close to 100°F and the sun of the California desert was baking my skin; I wanted to head back down. "OK, I've had enough, I'm coming down," I yelled out to my belay. He held firm on the rope and said, "Keep going up, you can do it!" "No," I yelled back, "I don't see any more handholds or footholds. I made it farther than I thought I would and I'm happy. I want to come down!" "You're rationalizing," my belay yelled up to me. "What else in your life do you rationalize about because you don't want to make the effort?"

"What are you, a psychotherapist?" I said, laughing. His replies were frustrating me, but part of me was also inspired by them.

Then he said something I will never forget: "Just raise yourself up on your tip toes and pull yourself up just a few inches, then a whole new set of possibilities may open up to you." I did what he suggested, and lo and behold, I saw another foothold, then a handhold. I was able to climb all the way to the top. It was exhilarating!

I realized then that it's not necessary to tackle everything in giant steps; no one climbs a mountain in one giant leap! Sometimes baby steps—putting just one foot in front (or above) the other—works perfectly. You'll get to your destination eventually. This bit of advice is so true in many areas in life, even when it comes to transforming your home and lifestyle to a cleaner, healthier one.

If you make just a few small super natural changes in your life using the ideas in this book, you can achieve more results than you ever thought possible.

So, I end this with three final suggestions, or 3 ways to make a shift, that will help make your transition to better health and greater vitality easier:

3 WAYS TO MAKE A SHIFT

1. Take the Super Natural Home Quiz again. See how much you've improved, then practice the ideas you've learned—everywhere, all the time, when-

ever you eat or drink, or put something on your skin, and when you travel.

2. Be an informed consumer. Check out the Recommended Resources beginning on page 192 to find more places to shop for nontoxic items for your home, plus books that may offer additional information and inspiration. Also, visit my Web site for updates on new super natural products as well as new research on health, home, and the environment: www.supernaturalhome.com.

3. Start from the inside out, beginning with your mind by keeping a positive attitude. Negative thoughts and emotions can be more harmful to our health and wellness than the toxins found in our homes. The good news is that we can produce natural healing chemicals in our bodies by focusing on love, faith, hope, joy, and gratitude. In the words of William James: "Human beings, by changing the inner attitudes of their minds, can change the outer aspects of their lives."

This book is my way of passing along my Grandma Bertha's message. My deepest wish is for each one of us to become intensely curious about our surroundings, start making smart choices to create a healthy home environment where we can all flourish. Greater vitality awaits you. Now go and make the right choices! Here is a summary of 10 easy ways to decrease the amount of chemical toxins you are exposed to on a daily basis. You will be healthier, your home will be transformed into a safe haven, and you will help create a healthier planet!

10 Easy Ways to Have a Super Natural Home

What Goes *in* You

1. Eat organic or pesticide-free foods whenever possible. Shop at farmers' markets or plant your own garden.

2. Read labels and avoid food additives such as MSG, trans fats (partially hydrogenated oils), and artificial sweeteners and artificial colors; they can cause behavioral and health problems.

3. Choose filtered tap water over bottled; it will have fewer bacteria and chemical contaminants. The bottled water industry is largely unregulated in the United States. Choose glass or stainless steel water containers.

What Goes *on* You

4. Use natural, chemical-free body care products and cosmetics with the fewest and safest ingredients. Watch out for parabens; they contain phthalates, known to interfere with our hormones.

5. Be cautious of any products with "fragrance," including shampoos, lotions, and perfumes. Pick those made with essential oils instead.

What *Surrounds* You

6. Clean your house with nontoxic natural cleaning products. Try vinegar, baking soda, and hydrogen peroxide. Avoid chlorine bleach, strong solvents, ammonia, and antibacterial products made with triclosan, as well as synthetically fragranced candles, laundry detergents, air fresheners, and dryer sheets.

7. Avoid volatile organic compounds (VOCs), found in vinyl wallpaper and floor coverings, new carpeting, and paint.

8. Sleep on a mattress made from untreated, nontoxic natural materials. If you can't afford a new mattress, buy a wool and organic cotton mattress topper. Natural mattresses are sold at JCPenney and IKEA.

9. Switch to sheets and towels made with bamboo or organic cotton. Regular cotton is one of the most intensively sprayed crops in the world. By some estimates, cotton accounts for 25% of all pesticides used in the United States. Macy's and Pottery Barn now sell organic cotton.

10. Get rid of nonstick, Teflon cooking pans; they emit potentially toxic fumes when heated. Use cast-iron, stainless steel, enamel, or glass cookware.

Supporting Information

RECOMMENDED RESOURCES

"Know where to find the information and how to use it—that's the secret of success."

—ALBERT EINSTEIN

The following is a listing of recommended books, Web sites, organizations, additional information, and other trusted resources to help you live a more Super Natural life. This guide is by no means complete. It would be impossible to list every resource available to you, which is why I invite you to explore options in your local area. Also go to www.supernaturalhome.com for updated information and help in finding the best products to support your journey to overall health and well-being.

WHAT GOES *IN* YOU

Books

Animal, Vegetable, Miracle by Barbara Kingsglover (Harper Collins, 2007)

Bottomfeeder: How to Eat Ethically in a World of Vanishing Seafood by Taras Grescoe, (Bloomsbury USA, 2008)

A Consumer Dictionary of Food Additives by Ruth Winter (Three Rivers Press, 2004)— offers the derivation and safety of most food additives (note: a new edition will be out April 2009)

The Encyclopedia of Natural Medicine by Michael Murray and Joseph Pizzorno (Three Rivers Press, 1997)

The End of Food by Paul Roberts, (Houghton Mifflin, 2008)

Excitotoxins: The Taste that Kills by Russell Blaylock, (Health Press, 1996)

Exposed: The Toxic Chemistry of Everyday Products and What's at Stake for American Power, by Mark Schapiro (Chelsea Green, 2007)

Fast Food Nation by Eric Schlosser (Houghton Mifflin, 2001)

Grub: Ideas for an Urban Organic Kitchen by Anna Lappe (Tarcher, 2006)

The Hidden Messages in Water by Masaru Emoto (Atria, 2005)

In Defense of Food by Michael Pollan (Penguin, 2008)

The Maker's Diet by Jordan Rubin (Siloam, 2004)

Nourishing Traditions by Sally Fallon (New Trends Publishing, 2001)

The Omnivore's Dilemma by Michael Pollan (Penguin, 2006)

Organic, Inc by Samuel Fromartz (Harvest Books, 2007)

Silent Spring by Rachel Carson (released in 1962; Marinar Books, 2002)

Pasture Perfect by Jo Robinson (Vashon Island Press, 2004)

The Slow Poisoning of America by John Erb, (Paladins Press, 2003)

What to Eat by Marion Nestle (North Point Press, 2006)

Web Sites

Find a farmer's market: www.ams.usda.gov/farmersmarkets

Find restaurants serving locally grown food: www.chefscollaborative.org

Genetically modified organism food listing: www.dadamo.com/frankenbase/list.cgi

Get better food into your kids' schools: www.farmtoschool.org

Information on ingredients and additives in your favorite brand-name packaged foods: www.labelwatch.com

Join a community garden: www.communitygarden.org

Learn more about the slow food movement: www.slowfoodusa.org

List of safe seafood choices: www.oceansalive.org

Food Blogs

Ban Trans Fats: www.bantransfats.com

ChewsWise: Digesting the Sustainable Food Chain: www.chewswise.com

Culinate: www.culinate.com

The Daily Table: www.sustainabletable.org/blog

Eating Liberally: www.eatingliberally.org

Eat Local Challenge: www.eatlocalchallenge.com

Edible Nation: www.ediblecommunities.com/ediblenation/

Edible Schoolyard Program: www.edibleschoolyard.org

Farm to School Program: www.farmtoschool.org

Food & Water Watch: www.foodandwaterwatch.org

Mighty Foods: www.mightyfoods.com

Slow Food Nation: www.slowfoodnation.org

What to Eat: www.whattoeatbook.com

Food Documentaries

Flow, by Irena Salina: www.flowthefilm.com

Food Fight, by Chris Taylor: www.foodfightthedoc.com

The Future of Food, by Deborah Koons Garcia: www.thefutureoffood.com

King Corn, by Ian Cheney: www.kingcorn.net

Mail-Order Organic Foods

Blackwing, Inc.: www.blackwing.com

Delicious Organics: www.deliciousorganics.com

Diamond Organics: www.diamondorganics.com

Papa's Organic: www.papasorganic.com

Transition Nutrition: www.transitionnutrition.com

Vital Choice Wild Seafood & Organics: www.vitalchoice.com

Wilderness Family Naturals: www.wildernessfamilynaturals.com

Additional Information on Food Additives

According to the Center for Science in the Public Interest, these food additives are unsafe in the amounts consumed or are very poorly tested and should be avoided:

Olestra (Olean)   **Potassium bromate**   **Propyl gallate**

Sulfites

Used primarily to reduce or prevent spoilage and discoloration, sulfites can trigger severe allergic reactions, especially in people with asthma. Since the FDA considers this additive to be safe, it is up to you to avoid it if you think you have a sensitivity. Sulfites appear on package labels as sulfur dioxide, sodium sulfite, sodium and potassium bisulfite, and sodium and potassium metabisulfite. Sulfites are frequently used in salad bars without notification of the consumer. Sulfites are commonly found in:

Corn syrup	Packaged lemon juice	Shellfish
Dried fruits	Salad dressings	Soups
Maraschino cherries	Sauces and gravies	Wine vinegar

Nitrates

Nitrates are added to about 60 percent of all pork produced in the United States. They are found in processed meats such as bacon, sausage, luncheon meats, and hot dogs.

Barcodes

The following numeric codes indicate where a product has been made:

00–13 US and Canada	57 Denmark	480 Philippines
30–37 France	64 Finland	628 Saudi Arabia
40–44 Germany	76 Switzerland and	629 United Arab Emirates
49 Japan	Liechtenstein	690–695 China
50 United Kingdom	471 Taiwan	740–745 Central America

Water Filter Guide

The National Geographic GreenGuide has published a brand-specific inquiry into the effectiveness of various water filters: www.thegreenguide.com

The Natural Resources Defense Council (NRDC) has a consumer guide to water filters that describes common filtration technology: www.nrdc.org

Water Filtration Systems

Consumer Reports: www.consumerreports.com

Heartspring: www.heartspring.net

Nikken: www.nikken.com

Omni Water Filters: www.omni-water-filters.com

Radiant Life Biocompatible Water System: www. radiantlifecatalog.com

Water Testing Lab

National Testing Laboratories: www. ntllabs.com

Shower Filters

New Wave Enviro: www.newwaveenviro.com

ZetaCore: www.carefreewater.com

For more information on the impact of plastic water bottles:

www.bottledwaterblues.com

www.reusablebags.com

More Facts about Water from the award-winning film Flow
www.flowthefilm.org

Of the 6 billion people on earth, 1.1 billion do not have access to safe, clean drinking water. (www.charitywater.org)

The U.S. Environmental Protection Agency currently does not regulate 51 known water contaminants. (www.foodandwaterwatch.org)

While the average American uses 150 gallons of water per day, those in developing countries cannot find five. (www.charitywater.org)

The water and sanitation crisis claims more lives through disease than any war claims through guns. (www.water.org)

According to the National Resources Defense Council, in a scientific study in which more than 1,000 bottles of 103 brands of water were tested, about one-third of the bottles contained synthetic organic chemicals, bacteria, and arsenic. (www.nrdc.org)

Water is a $400 billion dollar global industry, the third largest behind electricity and oil.

An estimated 500,000 to 7 million people in the United States get sick per year from drinking tap water.

California's water supply is running out—there is about 20 years of water left in the state. Maude Barlow, author of *Blue Covenant*, coauthor of *Blue Gold*.

Over 116,000 human-made chemicals are finding their way into public water supply systems. William Marks, author of *Water Voices from Around the World*.

In Bolivia, nearly one of every 10 children will die before the age of 5. Most of those deaths are related to illnesses that come from a lack of clean drinking water.

The cost per person per year for having 10 liters of safe drinking water every day is just $2 USD. Ashok Gadgil, Senior Staff Scientist in the Lawrence Berkeley National Laboratory.

WHAT GOES *ON* YOU

Books

Essence and Alchemy: A Natural History of Perfume by Mandy Aftel (Gibbs Smith, 2004)

Gorgeously Green by Sophie Uliano (Collins, 2008)

Healthy Child Healthy World by Christopher Gavigan (Dutton, 2008)

Not Just a Pretty Face by Stacy Malkan (New Society Publishers, 2007)

The Toxic Sandbox by Libby McDonald (Perigee Trade, 2007)

Web Sites

Campaign for Safe Cosmetics: www.safecosmetics.org

Cosmetic safety database by Environmental Working Group: Skin Deep: www.cosmeticsdatabase.com

Nanotechnology information: www.nanotechproject.org

Scorecard (run by the Environmental Defense Fund): www.scorecard.org

Natural Body Care Product Companies

Aubrey Organics: www.aubrey-organics.com

Cosmetics without Synthetics: www.allnaturalcosmetics.com

Lotus Moon: www.smbessentials.com

Made from Earth: www.madefromearth.com

Miessence Certified Organic Skin Care: www.micozyliving.com

MyChelle Dermaceuticals: www.mychelleusa.com

Pangea Organics: www.pangeaorganics.com

PeaceKeeper Cause-metics: www.Iamapeacekeeper.com

Perfect Organics: www.perfectorganics.com

Pharmacopia: www.pharmacopia.com

Revolution Organics: www.revolutionorganics.com

Tropical Traditions (coconut oil–based products): www.tropicaltraditions.com

Other Chemicals to Avoid in Cosmetics and Personal Care Products

DEA (diethanolamine), MEA (monoethanolamine), TEA (triethanolamine): found in products that foam, including bubble baths, body washes, shampoos, soaps, and facial cleaners.

FD & C color pigments: these can be made from coal tar, which is carcinogenic.

Fragrance: found in deodorants, shampoos, sunscreen, and baby products; most fragrances are synthetic, are made from petrochemicals, and contain phthalates.

Hydroquinone: found in skin-lightening creams.

Nanoparticles: found in skin cream, sunscreen.

Petroleum byproducts: mineral oil, paraffin, and petrolatum; baby oil is 100% mineral oil.

Phenol carbolic acid: found in lotions and skin creams.

Polyethylene glycol (PEG): found in cleansers.

Propylene glycol (PG): penetration enhancer, found in stick deodorants, body wash, acne treatment.

Sodium lauryl (or laurel) sulfate (SLS) and sodium laureth sulfate (SLES): penetration enhancer, sometimes disguised with the labeling "comes from coconut" or "coconut-derived"; found in shampoo/conditioner, liquid hand soap, shaving products.

Talc: found in blush, powder eye shadow, baby powder.

Triclosan: found in antibacterial soaps and toothpaste.

WHAT *SURROUNDS* YOU

Books

Big Green Purse by Diane MacEachern (Penguin, 2008)

The Body Toxic by Nena Baker (North Point Press, 2008)

Home Design with Feng Shui by Terah Kathryn Collins, (Hay House, 1999)

Home Safe Home by Debra Lynn Dadd (Tarcher/Penguin, 2005)

The Hundred-Year Lie by Randall Fitzgerald (Plume, 2006)

The Naturally Clean Home by Karyn Siegel-Maier (Storey, 1999)

Secret History of the War on Cancer by Devra Davis (Basic Books, 2007)

Web Sites

Children's Health Environmental Coalition: www.checnet.org

Childsake: www.childsake.com (children's environmental books)

Collaborative on Health and the Environment: www.healthandenvironment.org

The Daily Green: www.thedailygreen.com

Detoxics: www.detoxics.org

Environmental Health News: www.environmentalhealthnews.org

Environmental Research Foundation: www.rachel.org

The Green Guide: www.thegreenguide.com (reviews potentially dangerous chemicals found in household cleaning products)

The Green Seal Program: www.greenseal.org (provides certification standards for environmentally safe products)

Greenpeace: www.greenpeace.org

Health and Environment: www.healthandenvironment.org

Healthy Child: www.healthychild.org

To find a collection site for disposing of hazardous household products: www.earth911.org.

Bedding, Furniture, Home Interior, and Green Building Resources

E3 Environmental: www.h3environmental.com (Mary Cordaro's Web site)

Eco-conscious home and outdoor products: www.gaiam.com

Ecohaus: www.environmentalhomecenter.com

Eco Nest: www.econest.com (healthy home building)

Geo Swan: www.geoswan.com (green home building)

Green Home: www.greenhome.com

Healthy Building: www.healthybuilding.net

Natura Bed Systems: www.nontoxic.com/natura

Natural bedding, furniture, toys: www.ecochoices.com

Online source for green home products: www.healthyhome.com

Product reviews: www.healthyhouseinstitute.com

Air Purifiers

Air Purifiers America: www.air-purifiers-america.com

Clear Flite Air Purifiers: www.airpurifiers.com

Personal Air Purifiers: www.weinproducts.com

Pionair: www.pionair.net

Ultra-Pure Air Purifiers: www.ultra-pureair.com

EMF Reducers

Cutting Edge Catalog: www.cutcat.com

Less EMF Catalog: www.lessemf.com

Resources on Environmental Pollutants

Agency for Toxic Substances and Disease Registry: www.atsdr.cdc.gov (information about exposure and what toxins do)

Environmental Health Advocacy: www.healthybuilding.net

Environmental Protection Agency's Aging Initiative: www.epa.gov/aging (offers information on household and environmental hazards for older Americans)

Green California: www.green.ca.gov (provides reference materials and information on environmentally friendly products and services)

Green Guide: www.thegreenguide.com (reviews potentially dangerous chemicals found in household items)

Health effects of chemicals and fragrances in health care: www.massnurses.org/health

Household products database: www.householdproducts.nlm.nih.gov

Multiple Chemical Sensitivity (MCS): http://nofragrance.org

National Cancer Institute Fact Sheet "Formaldehyde and Cancer: Questions and Answers": www.cancer.gov/cancertopics/factsheet/Risk/formaldehyde

Strategic solutions for green chemicals: www.safer-products.org

Toxic chemicals in our environment: www.scorecard.org

For information about biological pollutants, combustion pollutants, asbestos, and indoor air quality in your home, write to: U.S. Consumer Product Safety Commission, Washington, DC 20207; 800-638-2772; www.cpsc.gov

Other Environmental websites

Air quality index and information: www.airnow.gov

Allergy Buyers Club: www.allergybuyersclub.com (products for those with sensitivities)

Chemical industry archives: www.chemicalindustryarchives.org (a project of the Environmental Working Group)

Environmental Health Perspectives: www.ehponline.org (free online publication reporting research and news on the impact of the environment on human health)

National Agricultural Statistics Service, database of agricultural chemical use: www.pestmanagement.info

Natural Resources Defense Council: www.nrdc.org

Pesticide Action Network North America: www.panna.org

Pesticide Action Network, pesticide database: www.pesticideinfo.org (for current toxicity and regulatory information for pesticides)

Right-to-Know Network: www.rtknet.org (provides free access to numerous databases and resources on the environment)

US Geological Survey's Pesticide National Synthesis Project: http://water.usgs.gov

Nontoxic Cleaning Supplies

Daddy Van's (beeswax furniture polish): www.daddyvans.com

Dr. Bronner's Magic Soaps: www.drbronner.com

Earth Friendly Products: www.ecos.com

Lily's Garden Herbals: www.lilysgardenherbals.com

Lucky Earth Products: www.luckyearth.com

Moon Works: www.moonworls.com

North Star Natural Pet Products: www.northstarpetsonline.com

Seaside Naturals: www.seasidenaturals.com

Seventh Generation: www.seventhgeneration.com

Organic Aromatherapy Essential Oils and Dried Herbs

Aroma Vera: www.aromavera.com

The Essential Oil Company: www.essentialoil.com

Mia Rose: www.miarose.com

Mountain Rose Herbs: www.mountainroseherbs.com

Organic and wild-crafted essential oils: www.naturesgift.com

SunRose Aromatics: www.sunrosearomatics.com

White Lotus Aromatics: www.whitelotusaromatics.com

Toxic Chemicals Typically Found in Your Home

Researchers name 216 chemicals that cause breast cancer in animal tests. Here are some of the most widespread:

Chemical	Source/use
1,4-dioxane	Detergents, shampoos, soaps
1,3-butadiene	Common air pollutant; found in vehicle exhaust
Acrylamide	Fried foods
Benzene	Common air pollutant; found in vehicle exhaust
Perfluorooctanoic acid	Used in manufacture of Teflon
Styrene	Used in manufacture of plastics; found in carpets, adhesives, hobby supplies, and other consumer products
Vinyl chloride	Used almost exclusively by the plastics industry to make vinyl
1,1-dichloroethane	Industrial solvent; also found in some consumer products, such as paint removers
Toluene diisocyanate	Used in foam cushions, furnishings, bedding
Methylene chloride	Used in furniture polish, fabric cleaners, wood sealants, and many other consumer products
Polychlorinated biphenyls (PCBs)	Electrical transformers; banned but still in environment
Polycyclic aromatic hydrocarbons (PAHs)	Diesel and gasoline exhaust
Atrazine	Widely used herbicide, particularly for corn

Source: Silent Spring Institute

Additional chemicals found in household disinfectants

- Formaldehyde, found in spray and wick deodorizers, which is a suspected carcinogen
- Petroleum solvents in floor cleaners may damage mucous membranes
- Butyl cellosolve, found in many all-purpose and window cleaners, may damage your kidneys, bone marrow, liver and nervous system
- Triclosan, the active ingredient in most antibacterial products, not only kills bacteria, it also has been shown to kill human cells

AWAY FROM HOME

To Learn More about Food Service in Hospitals

American Hospital Association: www.aha.org

American Society for Healthcare Food Service Administrators: www.ashfsa.org

National Society for Healthcare Foodservice Management: www.hfm.org

50 Best Ecotourism Lodges in the World

http://adventure.nationalgeographic.com

Tips for Greener Travel from the Green Hotels Association

BEFORE YOU LEAVE HOME

- Turn water heater to "Vacation" or lowest setting.
- Turn off AC/heat or adjust the thermostat to protect plants, etc.
- Appliances, such as TVs and cable converter boxes, should be unplugged because they can draw or "leak" as much as 40 watts per hour even when they're off.

TRAVEL

- Purchase electronic tickets for airline travel whenever possible (less waste). If paper tickets are lost, they may cost $75–$100 to be replaced.
- Use public transportation when available.
- Use the hotel van instead of renting a car.
- Take photos with a digital camera. Disposable cameras are very wasteful and expensive.

HOTEL STAYS

- Participate in hotel linen programs, or let the hotel know that it's not necessary to change your sheets and towels every day.
- When you leave your hotel room, turn off the AC/heat, lights, TV, and radio. Close the drapes.
- Leave little bottles of amenities in the guestroom if unopened.
- Check out of the hotel via the hotel's electronic program, available on the TV in some hotels, to reduce paperwork.

FOOD/RESTAURANTS

- Carry bottled water with you, preferably in a stainless steel container.
- Bring a small container—they come in handy for saving half-eaten treats or restaurant leftovers.
- Avoid Styrofoam; carry your own cup.

LIFESTYLE AND HEALTH

Books

Ageless Body Timeless Mind by Deepak Chopra (Harmony, 1994)

Micro-Miracles by Dr. Ellen Cutler (Rodale, 2005)

Perfect Health by Deepak Chopra (Harmony, 1991)

Raising Children Toxic Free by Philip Landrigan, MD (Farrar Straus Giroux, 1994)

Spontaneous Healing by Andrew Weil (Ballantine, 2000)

You: Staying Young by Michael Roizen and Mehmet Oz (Free Press, 2007)

Health Education

Dr. Mercola's Optimal Wellness Newsletter: www.mercola.com

Institute for Functional Medicine: www.functionalmedicine.org

Natural News: www.naturalnews.com

Weston A. Price Foundation: www.westonaprice.org

Personal Growth Education

The Hoffman Institute: www.hoffmaninstitute.org (An educational organization dedicated to restoring integrity, balance, and wholeness to people. Its Quadrinity Process, integrating the spirit, emotions, intellect, and physical body, is an 8-day residential program designed to eliminate unproductive, self-sabotaging patterns of feeling, thinking, and behaving.)

Detoxification Books

Detox Strategy by Brenda Watson (Free Press, 2008)

Detoxify or Die by Sherry Rogers (Prestige, 2002)

Live Free from Asthma and Allergies by Dr. Ellen Cutler (Celestial Arts, 2007)

Our Toxic World by Doris Rapp (Environmental Research Foundation, 2003)

Toxic Overload by Paula Baillie-Hamilton (Avery, 2005)

Toxicity-Testing Laboratories

Accu-Chem Laboratories: www.accuchem.com

Genova Diagnostics: www.gsdl.com

Immunosciences Lab: www.immuno-sci-lab.com

Detoxification Programs and Centers

BioSET: www.bioset.net (Dr. Ellen Cutler, Bioenergetic Sensitivity and Enzyme Therapy)

Core Care Center: www.corecarecenter.com (Marc Weill)

Hippocrates Health Institute: www.hippocratesinst.com

Optimum Health Institute: www.optimumhealth.org

Lifestyle Product Web Sites

Bamboo baby products—Bamboosa: www.bamboosa.com

Design Sponge: www.designspongeonline.com

Eco-conscious clothing, wellness, and beauty products: www.clarysageorganics.com

Eco-Fabulous: ecofabulous.blogs.com

Green and socially conscience fashion launched by Bono: www.edunonline.com

Green Plants for Green Buildings: http://greenplantsforgreenbuildings.org

Handcrafted, organic, home, and clothing (VivaTerra): www.vivaterra.com

How-tos and product reviews for sustainable living: www.sustainlane.com

Natural air fresheners: www.elizabethmorgan.net (try White Fire Purifying Room Spray)

Nontoxic Toys: www.achildsdream.com

Organic clothing: www.underthecanopy.com

Organic cotton and hemp collars for dogs and cats, as well as leashes, harnesses, and dog toys: www.thegooddogcompany.com

Organic flowers, plants, and chocolates: www.organicbouquet.com

Organic kid's clothing: www.gardenkids.com

Organic kids clothing and playthings: www.underthenile.com

Target's line of organic kids clothes, Under the Canopy: www.target.com

Log onto www.supernaturalhome.com for updates on natural products.

GLOSSARY

AEROSOL: A pressurized mist or spray containing minute particles used in self-dispensing products for the home.

ARTIFICIAL COLORS: Colors that can be used in foods, drugs, and cosmetics (known as FD&C colors). These are usually made from coal tar. "Natural" foods, such as oranges and farmed salmon, are sometimes dyed with artificial colors to make them more appealing. Artificial colors have been shown to aggravate symptoms of attention-deficit and attention-deficit hyperactivity disorders in children.

BAU-BIOLOGIE (BUILDING BIOLOGY): The study of how buildings affect our health.

BLOOD–BRAIN BARRIER: A filtering mechanism of the capillaries that carry blood to the brain and spinal cord tissue, blocking the passage of certain substances and preventing the accumulation of toxins that cause brain damage. Some toxic chemicals can cross this barrier.

BODY BURDEN (BIOACCUMULATION, CHEMICAL LOAD): The amount of harmful chemicals and pollutants found in a person's blood; describing substances that build up in the body faster than the body can eliminate them.

CARCINOGEN: A substance capable of producing cancer in living tissue.

CHEMICAL SENSITIVITY (MULTIPLE CHEMICAL SENSITIVITY [MCS]): An inability to tolerate, or extreme sensitivity or allergic reaction to, any of various chemical compounds present in everyday environments. MCS often results from prolonged exposure to chemicals.

CHRONIC TOXICITY: The slow or delayed onset of an adverse effect, usually from multiple, long-term exposures to toxins.

COAL TAR: An extract of coal used in the manufacture of dyes, cosmetics, and synthetic flavoring extracts. The EPA says it's highly toxic to humans.

CUMULATIVE EFFECT: What occurs from repeated exposures over time. This can be exposure to a small amount of one chemical over time, or exposure to multiple chemicals in a short amount of time.

DETOXIFICATION: The process of removing toxins from the body.

EMFs AND EMR: Electromagnetic fields and electromagnetic radiation. They are created by electric current and transport electric as well as magnetic energy. They play an important role in regulating bodily functions. The most common sources include high-voltage power lines, house wiring, and household appliances.

ENDOCRINE DISRUPTORS: Chemicals that can block the production of the male sex hormone testosterone, mimic the action of the female sex hormone estrogen, and interfere with the thyroid hormone.

ENVIRONMENTAL ILLNESS (EI): An increased sensitivity to chemicals and other irritants found in the environment.

EPA: Environmental Protection Agency, an agency of the federal government of the United States charged with protecting human health and with safeguarding the natural environment.

FACTORY FARMING OR CAFOs (CONFINED ANIMAL FEEDING OPERATIONS): The practice of raising farm animals and fish in confinement where a farm operates as a factory. There is lack of natural vegetation that the animals can eat, and pollution is produced from the animal waste.

FLAME RETARDANTS (BROMINATED FLAME RETARDANTS): Chemicals applied to electronics, clothes, and furniture to prevent them from catching fire. They are found in polar bears and eagles, and in human breast milk, where they pass from mother to child. Studies have shown that they can be absorbed through the skin even from garments washed more than 50 times.

FOOD ADDITIVES: Substances intentionally added to food to preserve flavor or improve taste and appearance. According to the FDA, some 2,800 substances are currently added to foods; some are known to be carcinogenic or toxic. Hyperactivity in children, allergies, asthma, and migraines are often associated with adverse reactions to food additives.

FORMALDEHYDE: A suspected human carcinogen that may be a contributing factor in SIDS, sudden infant death syndrome.

FRAGRANCE: This word on a label can indicate the presence of up to 4,000 synthetic ingredients.

GM OR GMO (GENETICALLY MODIFIED ORGANISMS): A plant, animal, or organism whose genetic material has been altered by using genetic engineering techniques.

INDUSTRIAL ORGANIC: Foods produced without synthetic chemicals, but not necessarily less processed, more local, or easier on the animals than conventionally grown and produced food.

INERT INGREDIENT: Any ingredient other than an active ingredient. Many inert ingredients are poisonous. Sometimes the term "other" will be substituted for the term "inert."

MSDS: Material Safety Data Sheets. Manufacturers publish the hazards and safety precautions for chemicals used in their manufacturing process.

MUTAGEN: A chemical that can permanently change the genetic content of the mother's or father's reproductive cells, thereby affecting the offspring.

NANOTECHNOLOGY OR NANOTECH: A process with the ability to manipulate and control matter on an atomic and molecular scale. It deals with structures, or nano particles, that are 100 nanometers or smaller. This new technology raises concerns about the toxicity and environmental impact of nano materials.

OFF-GASSING OR OUT-GASSING: The constant release of fumes, often undetectable.

PBDEs: Polybrominated diphenyl ethers; see flame retardants.

Supporting Information

PESTICIDES, HERBICIDES, AND FUNGICIDES: Chemicals used to mitigate or repel pests such as bacteria, insects, mites, birds, rodents, and other organisms that affect food production.

PFOA AND PFOs: Perfluorinated compounds, also known as C8, used in the production of Teflon cookware as well as stain- and grease-proof items such as fast-food wrappers. These chemicals are found in the bodies of people around the world, and in relatively high concentrations even in Arctic wildlife.

PHTHALATES: Chemicals used to soften plastics such as PVC, and also found in cosmetics and body care products. Proven to be endocrine disruptors, creating reproductive and developmental problems.

PLASTICIZERS: Chemical additives used to make hard plastics such as PVC soft and pliable.

PVC (POLYVINYL CHLORIDE): Plastic used in wall covering, flooring, clothing, toys, and other products too numerous to name. PVC manufacturing and disposal via incineration produce deadly dioxins.

SUSTAINABILITY: Using, developing, and protecting social and natural resources in a manner that allows people to meet their current needs without compromising the ability of future generations to meet their needs.

SYNERGISTIC EFFECT OR SYNERGISM: An effect that occurs when two or more substances or chemicals have a more powerful effect when used together. One chemical can interact in ways that enhance, magnify, or worsen the effects of the second.

SYNTHETIC: Artificial, not natural; something that has been formulated in a chemical laboratory.

TERATOGEN: A substance that causes permanent damage to a baby's cells, or birth defects.

TOXIN: Poisonous substance. It harms life.

TRADE SECRETS: Information that companies keep secret from the general public. How a product is made or ingredients that go into it can be legally protected as a trade secret.

VOLATILE ORGANIC COMPOUND (VOC): A toxic chemical substance that easily evaporates or vaporizes, giving off fumes into the atmosphere. Choose products labeled "No-VOC" or "VOC-free."

GIVING BACK

"We make a living by what we get, but we make a life by what we give."

—WINSTON CHURCHILL

IN THE SPIRIT OF GIVING BACK, I am delighted to donate a portion of the author proceeds from Super Natural Home to the following two worthy charitable organizations.

Search for the Cause. Its purpose is to investigate how exposures in our daily lives increase the risk of cancer, reduce harmful environmental conditions, and educate communities on healthy lifestyle choices. The organization's goal is to search for the cause, seek solutions, and strive for healthy and sustainable communities.

Under its Teens Turning Green teen-led projects are two programs: Teens for Safe Cosmetics, which raises awareness and educates about potentially toxic chemicals that are present in daily-use products and advocates for policy change, and Teens for Healthy Schools, which focuses research on the products used on school campuses.

SEARCH FOR THE CAUSE
2330 Marinship Way, Suite 190, Sausalito, CA 94965
PO Box 1146 Ross, CA 94957 (mailing)
Phone: (415) 289-1001
Director: Judi Shils (judishils@earthlink.net)
Web site: **www.searchforthecause.org**

Healthy Child Healthy World. This organization is dedicated to protecting the health and well-being of children from harmful environmental exposures. HCHW educates parents, supports protective policies, and engages communities to make responsible decisions, simple everyday choices, and well-informed lifestyle improvements to create healthy environments where children and families can flourish. HCHW has become the nation's leading organization of its kind. They help millions of parents, educators, health professionals, and the general public take action to create healthy environments and embrace green, nontoxic steps.

HEALTHY CHILD HEALTHY WORLD
12300 Wilshire Boulevard, Suite 320
Los Angeles, California 90025
Phone: (310) 820-2030
Web site: www.healthychild.org

INDEX

Home environment
  eliminating toxic chemicals from
    in bedroom, 107–18
    in kitchen, laundry room, and
      bathroom, 148–63
    in living room, den, and home
      office, 119–35
  sources of pollution in, xvii, 104–6,
    121, 147
    health effects of, 119–20, 120
Home office. See Living room, den,
  and home office
Honey, uses for, 35, 36
Hormones
  endocrine disruptors and, 74, 79–80,
    90
  functions of, 74
Hospitals, 182–83
Hotels
  green, 174–75, 177
  ordering food in, xxxii, 171–72, 173
Household cleaners
  harsh, alternatives to, 150
  health problems linked to, 145, 146
  homemade, 150–52
  labeling of, 148, 148, 149, 152
  quiz about, xxxii
  safe, 148–49, 150, 157, 163–65,
    165, 190
  toxins in, 147
Household hazardous waste, disposing
  of, 151
Household products, artificially scented,
  xxviii
Houseplants, for air purification, 137,
  138
Hydrogen peroxide
  as bleach alternative, 153
  for household cleaning, 150, 151, 190
Hygiene hypothesis, 146

I

Immune system
  effect of cosmetics and body care
    products on, 70–71
  hygiene hypothesis and, 146
  supplement boosting, 173–74

Indoor air pollution, in home
  environment, xix, 104–6,
    121, 147
  health effects of, 119–20, 120
Infant care products, 97
Insect repellent, 104, 176
Ion generators, for purifying air, 136
Ionizers, electronic, for purifying air, 136

J

Jet lag, homeopathic remedy for, 173
Joseph, Stephen, 30, 185–86

K

Kid's room, quiz about, xxx
Kitchen
  controlling toxic exposure from, 3
  quiz about, xxvi–xxviii
  sources of pollution in
    household cleaners, 148–52
    lead glazes in dishware, 161–63
    nonstick cookware, 158–61

L

Labels. See Food labels; Product labels
Laundry detergents, 153–54
Laundry room, sources of pollution in,
  153–55
Lead
  in artificial turf, 181
  in dishware glazes, 161–63
  in lipstick, 83
  in toys, 116
Lemons, for preventing sickness from
  air travel, 174
Levin, Lisa, 101
Linens, bed and bath, 112–13
Linoleum, 124
Lipstick, lead in, 83
Living room, den, and home office
  quiz about, xxxi
  sources of pollution in, 119–21
    carpeting, 120–23
    floors, 123–25
    paint, 128–31

Plants, for air purification, _137_, _138_
Plastic bottles
  BPA in, xxviii, 61–62
  recycling numbers on, _67_
  for water
    alternatives to, 57, 62
    best choices of, 62–63, 65
    problems with, 59–61, 63
Plastic containers, chemicals leached
    from, xxviii
Plastic toys, 116
PLU number on produce, 51–52
Pollution, indoor air (see Indoor air
    pollution)
Popcorn
  nonorganic, pesticides in, _10_
  PFOA in packaging of, 160
Positive attitude, power of, 189
Potatoes, pesticides in, _17_
Potpourri, 156, 157
Poultry, growth hormones in, xxvi
Pregnancy, pesticides and, _8_
Price, Weston A., 36–39
Processed foods
  giving up, 2–3, 4
  MSG in, 25, 27
  trans fats in, 31–32, _31_
Produce. See Fruits; Vegetables
Product labels
  on body care products, _94_
  on cosmetics, 77
  on food (see Food labels)
  on household cleaners, 148, _148_,
    149, _152_
  on sunscreen, 97
Prostate cancer, from BPA in plastic,
    xxviii, 61
Puer tea, _18_
Purification, water, 58–59
Pur water system, 58
PVC
  dangers of, 126, 127
  in hospital flooring materials, _183_
  office supplies without, _134_
  in plastic bottles, 63, _67_
  in shower curtain liners, 125–26
  in toys, 116
  in vinyl wallpaper, xxix, 126

Q

Quiz, Super Natural Home, xx,
    xxv–xxxiii, 188–89

R

Radon, from granite countertops, _162_
rBGH (recombinant bovine growth
    hormone), in cow's milk, xxvi
Recipes
  for chicken nuggets, _32_
  for homemade sunscreens, 100
  for insect repellent, _176_
  for skin care products, 87
Recombinant bovine growth hormone,
    in cow's milk, xxvi
Recycling numbers on bottles, meaning
    of, _67_
Refrigerator, quiz about, xxvi–xxviii
Restaurant food. See also Restaurants
  for children, 172–73
  MSG in, 25, 27
  trans fats used in, xxxii, 28, 29, 31
Restaurants. See also Restaurant food
  conscious dining in, 170
  green practices of, _171_
Reverse osmosis water purification,
    58–59
Rice, genetically engineered, 49–50
Robinson, Jo, 18–19
Rostolder, Bertha, xvii, 189
Rugs. See also Carpeting
  Oriental, 123
  wool, 168

S

Salmon
  farm-raised, 47, _47_, 48, _48_
  genetically engineered, 53
Salt lamps, for improving air quality, 158
School(s)
  artificial turf and lead at, _181_
  eating at, 177–81, _179_, 184
Sea lice, from fish farms, 47, _47_
Shampoos, 90
Sheets, xxx, 112–13, 190